Sentiment Analysis in the Medical Domain

Kerstin Denecke

Sentiment Analysis in the Medical Domain

Springer

Kerstin Denecke
Bern University of Applied Sciences
Bern, Switzerland

ISBN 978-3-031-30186-5 ISBN 978-3-031-30187-2 (eBook)
https://doi.org/10.1007/978-3-031-30187-2

This Springer imprint is published by the registered company Springer Nature Switzerland AG
The registered company address is: Gewerbestrasse 11, 6330 Cham, Switzerland

Don’t let the lack of a perfect tool be the obstacle to reaching your goal. (Roger Penrose)

Preface

Sentiment analysis deals with extracting information about opinions, sentiments, and even emotions conveyed by writers towards topics of interest. Often, it is directly associated with analysing subjective texts such as customer reviews or tweets with the aim of studying the attitude of a writer towards a product or subject. However, sentiment analysis gained in interest also in the healthcare domain with multiple application areas. When publishing an overview paper on medical sentiment analysis in 2015 [49], I was thinking of the beginning of this research topic and envisioning first use cases in the clinical domain. Eight years later, some progress has been made in this field, even though it was less than expected: Methods for analysing sentiment are applied to (medical) social media data supporting researchers in learning more about diseases, perceptions, and needs of patients and their caregivers. Beyond, clinical narratives are increasingly used as subject of analysis by medical sentiment analysis methods. Recognising that clinical notes and other free-textual documents that are part of the electronic health record may contain valuable information, sentiment analysis results have been tested for predicting risks of developing mental diseases, for gathering patient-reported outcomes or for pharmacovigilance.

The primary purpose of this book is to provide the necessary background on medical sentiment analysis, ranging from a description of the notions of medical sentiment to use cases that have been considered already and application areas of relevance. It provides a comprehensive overview on existing methods of sentiment analysis applied to healthcare resources or health-related documents. I will describe the concrete challenges to be considered when developing sentiment analysis methods in the healthcare domain. At the end, I will conclude with open research avenues providing researchers indications which topics still have to be developed in more depth.

In more detail, the book is structured into four parts. In Part I, I define medical sentiment and give an overview on the various use cases that have been suggested and tested in the last years in research.

To conduct medical sentiment analysis, resources are required. In Part II, I describe available lexical resources, which are sentiment lexicons, but also textual resources. Medical sentiment analysis can be applied to clinical narratives or social media data. Even conversation protocols of chatbots can provide a source of analysis. These different text types and their characteristics will be described.

In Part III, I will provide an overview on existing medical sentiment analysis solutions. First, I summarise the levels and tasks that can be considered by medical sentiment analysis. Second, an overall overview on the different steps to pre-process documents is given. Third, the existing approaches to medical sentiment analysis are described. This part also introduces off-the-shelf tools that can be simply applied to a dataset to classify documents according to their sentiment or to analyse the polarity. Fourth, an outline of case studies provides concrete examples of how real-world problems can be solved with medical sentiment analysis.

In Part IV, I outline potential future directions within this research field. Thoughts on opportunities and challenges of bringing medical sentiment analysis into real-world applications will be described. Additionally, I will raise concerns related to unintended consequences and open challenges of this analysis. The book finishes with potential future research directions to move forward making this vision reality (vision was generated by ChatGPT in December 2022):

- *In the year 2040, the use of medical sentiment analysis will be widespread, as it becomes an integral part of healthcare, and is highly valued and respected.*
  It will be used to track trends and sentiment, and provide insights and guidance,
  To help healthcare professionals, deliver better care and support, to those in need, with precision and alliance.
  Medical sentiment analysis will be used to understand the emotions and experiences,
  Of patients and their families, and to identify areas for improvement and redress,
  It will be a valuable tool, for improving patient satisfaction and outcomes,
  And will be an essential part of healthcare, that is highly valued and in demand, without any doubts.

The Bern University of Applied Sciences supported this book project by funding a sabbatical which relieved me from teaching duties. I acknowledge collaboration and discussions with Yihan Deng about this topic. Parts of the book base upon a literature review conducted together with Daniel Reichenpfader. I would like to thank Frank Mathwig for his input on the unintended consequences of medical sentiment analysis. Last but not at least, I would like to thank my friends and colleagues for their encouragements and support on the various levels that writing a book requires.

Bern, Switzerland Kerstin Denecke
January 2023

Contents

Acronyms

ADE	Adverse Drug Event
ADR	Adverse Drug Reaction
AI	Artificial Intelligence
API	Application Programming Interface
CBT	Cognitive Behaviour Therapy
CNN	Convolutional Neural Network
ECG	Electrocardiogram
EHR	Electronic Health Record
FDA	Food and Drug Administration
i2B2	Informatics for Integrating Biology and the Bedside
ICU	Intensive Care Unit
LIWC	Linguistic Inquiry and Word Counts
MedRA	Medical Dictionary for Regulatory Analysis
MRI	Magnetic Resonance Imaging
NLP	Natural Language Processing
PREM	Patient-Reported Experience Measures
PROM	Patient-Reported Outcome Measures
RNN	Recursive Neural Network
SNOMED CT	Systematised Nomenclature of Medical Clinical Terms
SVM	Support Vector Machine
TF-IDF	Term Frequency-Inverse Document Frequency
TREC	Text Retrieval Conference
UMLS	Unified Medical Language System
VTE	Venous Thromboembolism
XAI	Explainable Artificial Intelligence

Part I
Landscape of Medical Sentiment

Chapter 1
What is Special about Medical Sentiment Analysis?

1.1 Overview

Research on sentiment analysis and opinion mining from reviews and social media became popular in 2004 [91] with use cases such as spam detection in social media [98], sentiment analysis in political debates [155], or analysis of customer reviews [68].

Medical sentiment analysis refers to the identification and analysis of sentiments or emotions expressed in free-textual documents with a scope on healthcare and medicine. It uses natural language processing (NLP), text analysis and machine learning to realise the process of extracting and classifying statements regarding expressed opinion and sentiment. Originating from the business and customer service domain [114], sentiment analysis methods are increasingly used in the medical domain to extract and classify information on clinical outcomes, to classify changes in the health status, or to judge automatically perceptions of treatments etc. Through an analysis of sentiments in medical social media, we can learn about the patient's attitude toward a doctor, and we gain knowledge on the patient's acceptance and satisfaction with a healthcare service. Most existing research on sentiment analysis in the medical domain concentrates on analysing patient opinions expressed in social media and in suicide notes [159].

In social media, patients or their relatives describe their perceptions and experiences with healthcare services or their experiences with treatments and living with diseases. Furthermore, they ask for help or discuss treatments or symptoms with others. Those patient-reported experiences and outcomes gain in interest in healthcare since they are providing valuable information on outcomes, efficacy of treatments and on health service quality [106]. It is time-consuming to manually process and analyse large volumes of social media text or forum postings. Sentiment analysis methods can support in this process.

In the context of healthcare, a broad range of free-textual documents reflects a patient's health status or the care process and delivers information on treatment

K. Denecke, *Sentiment Analysis in the Medical Domain*,
https://doi.org/10.1007/978-3-031-30187-2_1

outcomes. These documents include various types of clinical narratives written by health professionals for clinical documentation purposes such as discharge summaries, radiology reports or nursing notes. Even though written in an objective manner, those texts are increasingly recognised as important source of information for predicting risks and outcomes. In particular nursing notes can provide essential information on changes in the health status of a patient. Applying sentiment analysis to these documents can help in discovering those changes or risk factors.

Research already started to apply sentiment analysis methods to clinical narratives such as nursing notes [198], radiology reports [49] or discharge summaries [127]. By using sentiment analysis techniques on such document types, risks can be predicted or their results can provide more information about the health status of patients. It is still unknown whether analysing or taking into account these subjective attitudes may have an impact on diagnosing, accuracy of diagnoses or risk prediction because it is an active research area that has not yet been well established in software solutions for the healthcare industry. The potential benefits of applying sentiment analysis to textual data from the healthcare sector will be shown in the remaining chapters of this book.

A first overview and vision paper on medical sentiment analysis was published in 2015 [49]. After systematically comparing word usage and sentiment distribution between clinical narratives (nursing notes, discharge summary, and radiology reports) and medical social media (medical-related blogs, drug reviews), Denecke and Deng concluded that off-the-shelf sentiment analysis tools are not ideal for analysing sentiment in medical documents [49]. From clinical narratives such as nursing notes or radiology reports it turned out to be significantly more difficult to predict sentiment than from social media data. This is due to the fact that relevant vocabularies differ from general-domain sentiment and words can change their meaning depending on the entire medical history (e.g. a reduction of blood sugar is good when it was too high before but bad, when it was already critical). Another reason is that the notions of medical sentiment are extremely diverse depending on the use case of sentiment analysis in the medical domain.

Therefore, there is a need for domain adaptation of sentiment analysis that includes a richer array of attributes than can typically be found in off-the-shelf tools. This book will outline the development of this research topic. Even though there is still a lot of research applying off-the-shelf tools for extracting and analysing sentiment from medical-related documents, we will see that there have been also specific algorithms developed that consider the peculiarities of the medical domain and textual data from this domain.

The research topic of medical sentiment analysis comprises four dimensions (see Fig. 1.1): Data dimension, use dimension, task dimension and technology dimension. This book is structured along these four dimensions. The data dimension describes the data from which medical sentiment can be identified. This includes online textual content such as forum texts or social media text, but also clinical narratives and conversations with intelligent agents integrated in a healthcare application. Data resources are outlined in more detail in Part II. Medical sentiment analysis is of interest for several use cases which I summarise under the use

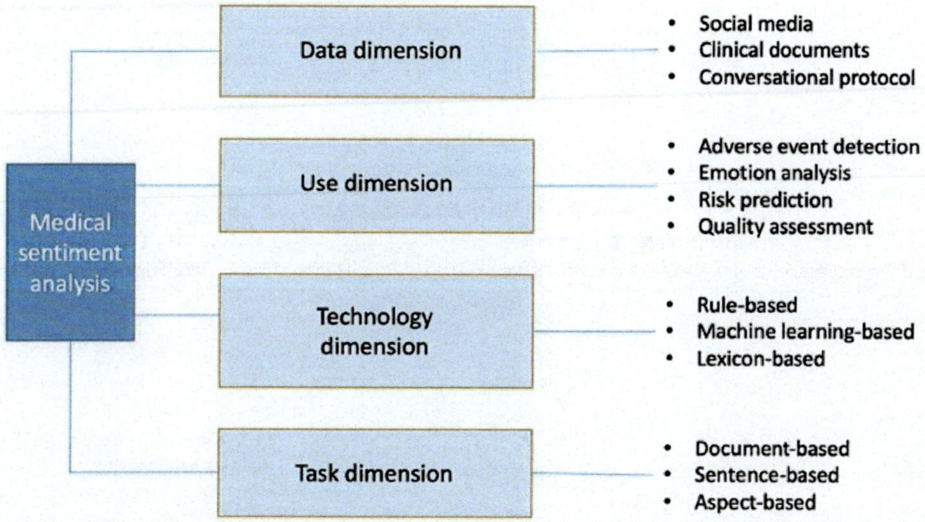

Fig. 1.1 Dimensions of the field of medical sentiment analysis: Roughly four dimensions can be distinguished. The book is structured along these dimensions

dimension (details in Chaps. 2 and 13). The task dimension considers the concrete task that is considered, i.e. whether sentiment is of relevance with respect to a specific aspect, for single sentences or overall for a document (see Chap. 8). Technology is needed to extract sentiments—this is summarised as technology dimension (see Part III of the book). This dimension includes algorithms, linguistic and lexical resources and off-the-shelf tools.

1.2 Opinion Definition

Medical sentiment analysis can be seen as a two-step process:

- **Health mention classification**: In this step, the topics of an input text are determined, i.e. which symptoms, diseases, treatments or other medical entities are mentioned towards which opinions are expressed. This step is also referred to as topic detection (see Sect. 9.6).
- **Sentiment analysis**: In this step, the sentiment is determined and analysed. This could be an emotion that is expressed or the polarity of the sentiment (e.g. positive or negative, neutral). It is associated to the identified health mention.

We will start with defining sentiment and opinion. In this book, I will adopt the definitions of the terms opinion and sentiment proposed by Liu [115] for the medical domain. According to his definition, an *opinion* is a quadruple comprising

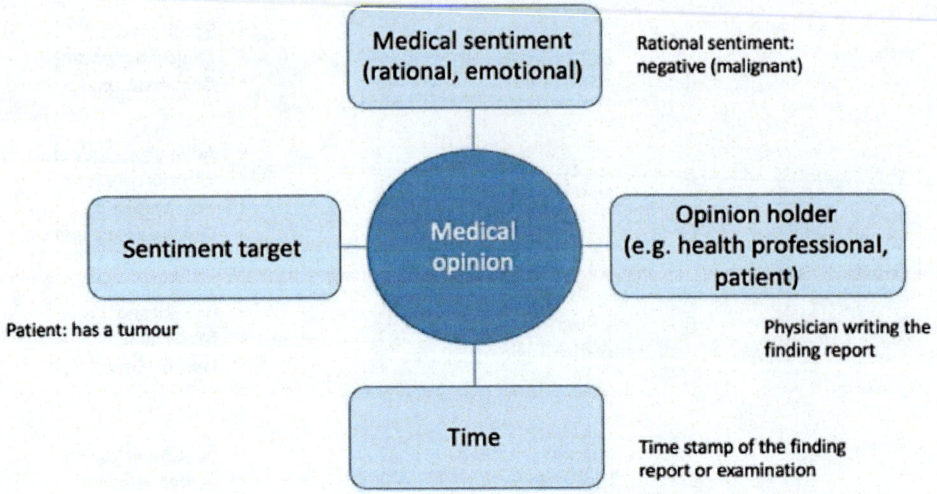

Fig. 1.2 Definition of medical opinion: It consists of a sentiment target, an opinion holder, a time and the sentiment. Consider the phrase "The tumour is malignant" which is a sentence from a finding report

- a *sentiment target*,
- a *sentiment* of the opinion about the target,
- an *opinion holder* and
- a *time* when the opinion was expressed.

The *sentiment target* is the entity on which a sentiment has been expressed upon [115]. As we will see in the use cases described in Chap. 2, medical sentiment can be expressed towards a diverse set of sentiment targets. A target can be seen as an attribute of a patient, a healthcare provider, a healthcare service (see Fig. 1.2). For example, a patient has an anatomical structure towards which an opinion is expressed; he has a health status, might have symptoms, receives a treatment, a diagnosis, shows a symptom in general or disease-specific risk factors etc. The *opinion holder* expresses the opinion through text. Concerning clinical narratives, the *opinion holder* expressing the opinion and *time* are only accessible from the overall document since it is normally written in passive voice.

Consider the following sentence from a finding report: *The remainder of the abdomen with and without Gadolinium is unremarkable.* The sentiment target is *The remainder of the abdomen*; the sentiment is represented by the term *unremarkable*; opinion holder and time are not mentioned explicitly, but we know, the document that contains this phrase has an author (the responsible physician) and a time stamp. In text passages that include indirect or direct speech, the opinion holder has to be identified. Medical sentiment and its notions are defined in more detail in the next section.

1.3 Definition of Medical Sentiment

A *medical sentiment* can be defined as an attitude, thought or judgement promoted by an observation with respect to the health of some individual [115, 147]. For medical sentiment, we can distinguish *rational sentiment* from *emotional sentiment* [115]. *Rational sentiments* originate from "rational reasoning, tangible beliefs and utilitarian attitudes. They express no emotions." [115]. An example would be the previously mentioned phrase "the tumour is malignant"—the phrase implies a rational sentiment (Fig. 1.2). *Emotional sentiments* originate from "non-tangible and emotional responses to entities which go deep into people's psychological state of mind" [115]. An example sentence expressing an emotional sentiment is "It was the worst pain I ever had".

Medical sentiment expresses judgements, vagueness, certainty etc. concerning a medical sentiment target (e.g. medical condition and its appearances and (health) consequences for an individual) [49]. Consider for example the following facets of sentiment in health-related texts [49]. Medical sentiment can concern (see Fig. 1.3):

- a change in the health status or behaviour (e.g. the health status of a patient can improve or get worse, or a patient can be compliant or non-compliant towards a treatment),
- critical events or situations that impact a patient's life (e.g. the statement "the tumour is malignant" as such is a fact, but this medical condition has negative implications for a patient since it might lead to health problems, treatments or even death),
- the outcome or effectiveness of a treatment (e.g. the outcome of a surgery can be good or bad),

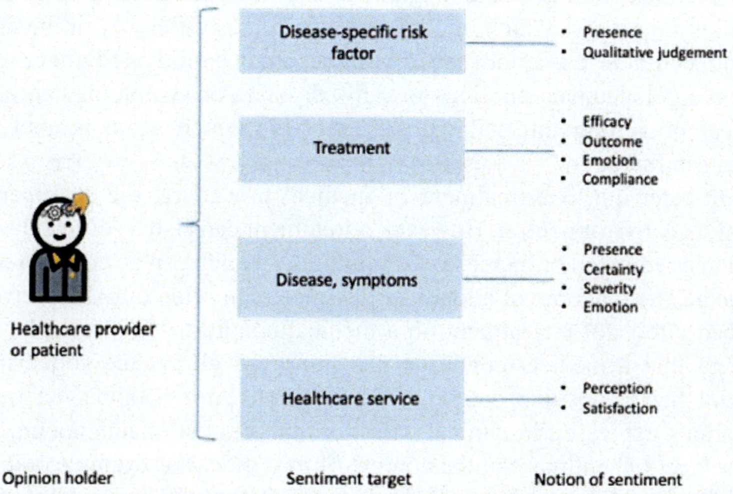

Fig. 1.3 Sentiment targets and notions of medical sentiment

- the certainty of a diagnosis (e.g. a physician may be certain or uncertain of some diagnosis),
- patient-reported experiences or outcomes towards a treatment or drug (e.g. a patient can describe serious adverse events after drug consumption or serious symptoms),
- feelings and emotions of daily life while suffering from a disease,
- absence or presence of a risk factor or a qualitative judgement (e.g. the patient's mental health status is described unstable or stable).

It might be necessary to concertise our general definition of medical sentiment and medical opinion for the medical speciality that is considered in a particular use case. Holderness et al. [87] provided a definition of the psychiatric clinical sentiment. Mapped to the previously introduced quadruple describing a medical opinion this means:

- *Opinion holder*: a clinician's attitudes which can be
- *Sentiment*: positive, negative, or neutral towards
- *Sentiment target:* a patient's prognosis with regard to seven readmission risk factor domains (appearance, mood, interpersonal relations, substance use, thought content, thought process and occupation). One sentiment per risk factor exists.

The psychiatric sentiment defined by Holderness comprises 7 sentiment targets, also referred to as risk factors. The time dimension remained unconsidered by Holderness et al. This concertised definition shows that medical sentiment can have multiple facets that depend on the considered aspect.

But not only the sentiment target can differ, also so sentiment can have multiple facets. A sentiment facet regarding a diagnosis, symptom or medical condition can concern the presence of these targets. It could concern the certainty of the opinion holder regarding the diagnosis. There are for example suspicions of a diagnosis mainly at the beginning of the diagnostic process or there are assured diagnoses at the end of the process which might be recognised as different sentiment notions. A symptom could have a certain severity: Pain could be mild, medium or severe. From a patient's perspective, emotions towards diseases or symptoms can be expressed (e.g. fear of getting infected with COVID-19) which again is another facet of medical sentiment.

When referring to a treatment or medical procedure, the sentiment might be positive, negative or neutral. However, a treatment can also be efficient or inefficient or lead to a reduction or increase of symptoms—which can be considered notions of sentiment. The outcome of a medical treatment can often only be derived from the described effects of a treatment on a medical condition. For example, a physician statement that a medical condition has improved allows the conclusion that the treatment had a positive outcome. Observations and opinions on treatments or medications expressed in clinical narratives or in social media documents provide another facet of sentiment in the context of medicine. For example, a drug can lead to a relief of pain. A treatment could be considered helpful by a patient (regardless of efficacy); the patient can be satisfied, which could be manifested in an achievement of personal health goals. A patient can be compliant with a certain treatment, e.g. taking the medications as prescribed or he/she can be non-compliant, ignoring the recommendations and prescriptions. Finally, medical sentiment can concern perceptions of the healthcare service quality, e.g. patient perceptions regarding the patient-doctor communication.

These examples demonstrate that medical opinions can be expressed towards a multitude of sentiment targets and that medical sentiment goes beyond the distinction of polarities. It becomes clear that the definition of medical sentiment depends on the use case and medical speciality. The base definition of medical opinion provided in this chapter provides guidance, but needs to be concertised for the considered health mention or health topic considered within the analysis.

Chapter 2
Use Cases of Medical Sentiment Analysis

2.1 Sentiment Analysis in Mental Health

Expressed opinions and choices of words—in online or in person discussions—are most of the times based on our sentiments. With the raise of social media, people started to express their sentiments and emotions on a regular basis and in written format. Analysing these sentiments from online discussions can help understanding the human behaviour. Mental health includes our emotional, psychological and social well-being and is therefore related to feelings, emotions and sentiments. Thus, it is obvious that one of the first applications of sentiment analysis in the health domain was related to mental health. It concerned the analysis of the risk of committing suicide based on data from online forums. A classifier that considered also the expressed sentiment of a text as feature was developed to differentiate suicidal and non-suicidal online posts [2]. This approach allowed to identify postings from people with suicidal ideation in online forums. From these postings, mental health researchers can learn more about these ideations, their progress and potential causes.

Detecting and diagnosing depressions normally rely on self-reporting of individuals in conjunction with informed assessment by healthcare professionals. Providing effective health monitoring systems and diagnostic tools could be useful to improve the work of healthcare professionals and reducing healthcare costs. Technology to capture feelings and emotions could help to achieve these goals by providing an objective assessment. Sentiment or even emotions expressed in tweets were successfully used (in conjunction with other features) as predictive features of major depressive disorder [196]. Even in combination with the analysis of facial expressions, sentiment analysis was tested in detecting depressions [140]. Because of the severity of the disease, side effects of treatments or death of other patients with the same disease, cancer patients tend to be affected by emotional disorders

K. Denecke, *Sentiment Analysis in the Medical Domain*,
https://doi.org/10.1007/978-3-031-30187-2_2

such as depression. Monitoring the mood of those patients—as sentiment analysis methods allow for—provides a means to identify risks of developing mental health diseases accompanying a cancer disease [166]. An early detection could support in providing help at an early stage of (mental) disease development.

Beyond analysing social media, also the sentiment analysis of unstructured data of the electronic health record (EHR), e.g. clinician's free-text notes and written records, may offer relevant information in the context of mental health. For example, care provider notes can be used to identify loneliness among the patients with existing mental health conditions [12]. Loneliness is characterised by negative feelings due to being alone which—ones documented by health providers in corresponding notes—can be detected with sentiment analysis.

Suicide risk can also be predicted from EHR data. In contrast to the previously described scenarios for social media, not the sentiment or emotion of a patient is explicitly analysed, but reflections or observations from nurses or physicians. Such data can reveal information about patients' interpersonal patterns [109]. Retrieving subjective clinical attitudes (sentiment) from clinical narratives was found to demonstrate potential to identify a worsening of symptoms or an increased readmission risk of psychotic patients [87]. Several risk factors (appearance, mood, interpersonal relationships, substance use, occupation, thought content, thought process) contribute to the psychiatric clinical sentiment. In this particular context, sentiment analysis is applied for classifying sentences or sequences of text that describe a certain risk factor as positive, neutral or negative. The integrated classification result for each risk factor domain can then be exploited in a classifier that predicts inpatient readmission risks [87]. Beyond classifying risk factors according to their polarity, methods of sentiment analysis can classify the severity of risk factors for developing or worsening mental diseases [167]. Figure 2.1 and Table 2.1 summarise use cases of medical sentiment analysis in the context of mental health.

2.2 Outcome and Quality Assessment of Healthcare Services and Technologies

Knowledge on the outcome and quality of healthcare services and health technologies can be gathered from clinical narratives stored in the EHR. However, also patient's experiences expressed in social media or as answers to open-ended questions in questionnaires provide such information. In this chapter, I present a few examples of information gathering from social media, patient surveys, and EHR data utilising medical sentiment analysis. Data resulting from such analysis is frequently employed to evaluate the effectiveness of healthcare interventions and services. Table 2.2 summarises the described use cases.

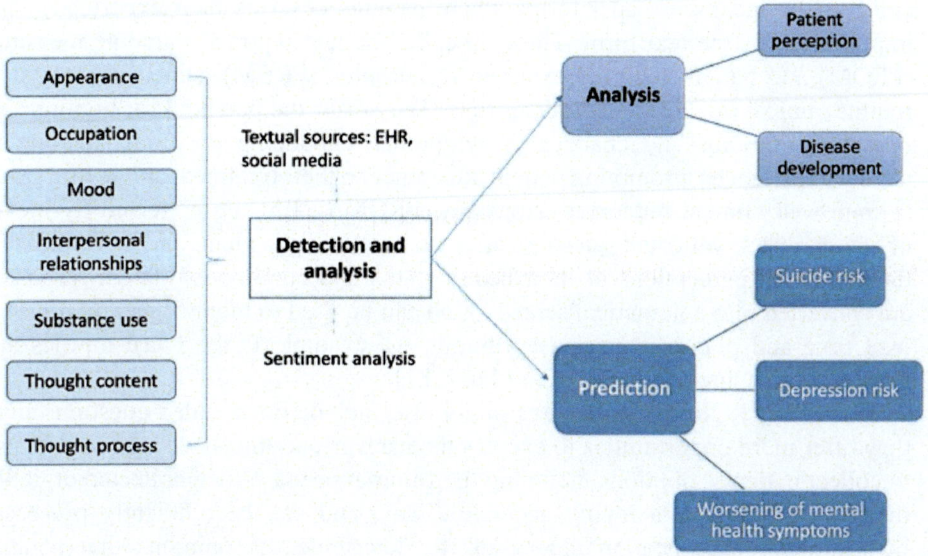

Fig. 2.1 Sentiment analysis and its use in mental health: Risk factors associated with mental diseases can be identified and analysed using sentiment analysis techniques from EHR data and social media data. The results can support prediction of mental health risks or in analysing patient perceptions and disease development

Table 2.1 Use cases in mental health—overview

Information need	Information on feelings and emotions of patients for the purpose of monitoring, prediction and analysis
Text sources	Social media, EHR
Example use case	Prediction of the psychiatric readmission risk, identification of suicide ideation, knowledge acquisition on mental diseases and patient perceptions

Table 2.2 Use cases for quality management—overview

Information need	Information on patient perceptions of consumed healthcare services, treatments or outcomes
Text sources	Social media, PROM/PREM questionnaires
Example use case	Analysis of free text comments in PROM questionnaires to learn more about subjective outcomes, analysis of healthcare service reviews to identify quality issues of an organisation, analysis of user reviews to understand reasons for non-adherence to digital health interventions

2.2.1 Analysis of Patient Questionnaires

For medical treatments which merely alleviate the symptoms of an illness or relieve pain, it is vital to discover the extent to which these are effective and what the actual impact on the patient's quality of life is. Feedback on those outcomes is often collected by means of paper forms where patients describe their experiences and impressions in free text form. These so-called patient reported outcome measures (PROM) and patient reported experience measures (PREM) gained in interest in routine clinical practice and clinical trials. They offer the potential for highlighting relevant symptoms and changes in symptoms, enhancing the understanding of patient experiences, promoting patient adherence to their treatment and in turn result in improved clinical outcomes. Normally, PROM/PREM are collected by means of standardised, validated questionnaires completed by patients trying to measure their personal perceptions of their health status and conditions. Patient responses are converted into a numerical score, which can be used to monitor patient progress over time and plan treatment accordingly. An example is the Knee injuries and Osteoarthritis Outcome Score as used in [181].

However, PROM questionnaires might also include open-ended questions since they offer more opportunities to express themselves and thus have a great potential to collect patients' opinions including their unmet needs. When collected digitally, the text is stored in a highly accessible way, and can be efficiently processed by sentiment classification algorithms to determine the opinions that patients are expressing [181]. In this particular use case, medical conditions, symptoms and other topics can be extracted together with a classification of the associated sentiment as expressed in the replies. This information enables health service provider to adapt their services accordingly, to identify quality issues [176] and to learn about clinical outcomes and their impact on patients.

2.2.2 *Clinical Outcome Analysis*

In addition to texts that are collected particularly for the purpose of quantifying patient reported outcomes, medical texts from routine care (i.e. EHR data) provide information on the treatment outcome. At the bedside, nurses and physicians reflect their observations which might become reported in clinical notes. Analysing these reflections with respect to sentiment can be useful for studying correlations, for example correlations between the intensive care unit (ICU) provider sentiment and the use of diagnostic imaging [70]. This helps in studying processes and the impact of attitudes and observations on decision making.

Sentiment analysis methods can be applied to distinguish no outcome, positive outcome, negative outcome, and neutral outcome [151] of treatments. Such analysis' findings aid in addressing research questions concerning an intervention's advantages and disadvantages. Finally, clinicians can get a basic impression of how "good" an intervention is based on the amount of positive or negative outcomes of an intervention applied to a disease.

Sentiment of clinical notes can also be considered in relation to changes over time, patient condition, and ethnicity [69]. This allows studying the impact of these aspects on the clinical outcome. Outcome as expressed by mortality and readmission can be studied. Correlations between sentiment expressed in clinical notes and these two aspects have been assessed already in some research [127, 198]. It can help in identifying quality issues that might contribute to negative outcomes.

2.2.3 Social Media as Mirror of Service Quality

Patients possess opinions about the healthcare services they receive. Each interaction with a care provider can trigger an emotional reaction. Sentiment analysis can help identifying and understanding these emotions. Insights that can be gained through analysing patient sentiments towards healthcare services can help optimising the patient experience. Different dimensions can be distinguished: system quality, interaction quality and information quality. By analysing feedback from patients using sentiment analysis, providers can examine whether patients feel well informed or whether there are drawbacks in patient-doctor/patient-nurse communication—just to mention a few examples.

Sentiments play an important role in patients' beliefs, attitudes and decisions and are often expressed in online reviews [173], but also in online surveys with open-ended questions. These reviews can concern different aspects regarding a healthcare provider such as service quality or satisfaction with healthcare service [76, 120, 173].

Assessing service quality of mobile healthcare services is of relevance for service providers [156]. From online health reviews, knowledge can be gained on how to improve healthcare service quality [202] or hospital service quality [102]. Once extracted, healthcare provider can learn from the negative comments, improve their service quality and in this way achieve increased economic returns [173]. Mammen et al. used a qualitative analysis to determine how patients and physicians perceive virtual visits for Parkinson's disease and to identify components contributing to positive and negative perceptions [124]. The data source were online surveys with five open-ended questions. The responses were analysed using sentiment analysis.

For instance, in 2021, a life science research team from Mount Sinai Hospital collected more than 30,000 online customer reviews from 500 hospitals and then performed an aspect-based analysis, comparing the hospitals according to four aspect-based ratings: doctors' services, staffs' services, hospital facilities and affordability. The result was a useful database that patients could easily peruse to compare and contrast their options. Additionally, it allowed hospital administrators to compare their facility against competitors in each of the four key categories, highlighting areas in which patient care may be improved.

Surveillance of social media platforms can provide relevant insights on the effectiveness and safety of the use of health technologies on a patient [161]. In the context of drugs, this is referred to as pharmacovigilance (see section below). However, it is of equal importance to study emotions and sentiment expressed towards mHealth apps since they become more popular and in some European countries it is already possible to prescribe mHealth apps as digital health interventions. To avoid or overcome drop out rates or reduced adherence to digital health interventions, it is important to understand user opinions of available health apps beyond star ratings. An analysis of sentiment expressed in free text comments on such apps can provide knowledge for the development of future mhealth apps [65]. Such analysis of user reviews combined with a thematic analysis can reveal potentials and limitations of mHealth apps. Beyond, it can help in detecting safety hazards: Mummalaneni et al. exploit sentiment analysis to determine which words and phrases are indicators of defects in online reviews for automatically discover defects in the baby crib industry [146].

2.3 Sentiment Analysis for Clinical Risk Prediction

Clinical risk management focuses on reducing hazards and patient damage. For this, it is necessary to identify the hazards and comprehend the contributing factors. Lessons from (early identified) adverse events and poor outcomes can be used to ensure that countermeasures are put in place to lower risks and that actions are taken to prevent the recurrence of such hazards. An overview on the use cases is provided in Table 2.3.

One aspect of interest in clinical risk management concerns mortality and readmission risk. Physicians and nurses are in contact with patients every day and document their (subjective) observations in clinical notes. In particular nurses have consistently contact with the patients and recognise signs of changes in their health. Their observations and judgements are documented in their daily reportings. However, in daily practice this information can remain unconsidered in clinical decision making given a high time pressure and information overload. Medical sentiment analysis could support in exploiting this text resource as parameters for prediction purposes since such observations are often not immediately reflected in clinical parameters resulting from diagnostic technologies.

Risk prediction systems often use structured data from the EHR to calculate scores (e.g. sequential organ failure assessment (SOFA), simplified acute physiology score (SAPS)). Nevertheless, also the unstructured data contained in a EHR might be useful for risk prediction. Sentiment analysis as a method to analyse unstructured data can contribute identifying the attitudes or impressions of clinicians or nurses towards patients. Analysing the sentiment in nursing notes can provide an additional source of information for mortality prediction, e.g., for predicting the 30-day

Table 2.3 Use cases in clinical risk prediction—overview

Information need	Information on (even subtle) changes in the patient health that are not reflected in data from laboratory tests, radiological imaging or other examination data
Text sources	EHR, social media
Example use case	Identifying risk factors for developing cardiovascular diseases; predicting the 30-day mortality risk in sepsis patients

mortality risk in sepsis patients [210] or mortality in intensive care [198]. An early prediction of risks helps to ensure that countermeasures are taken in time.

Another use case concerns classifying the severity of risk factors for developing specific diseases using sentiment analysis. This information can then contribute to the early diagnosis as has been demonstrated in the context of diagnosing venous thromboembolism (VTE) [167]. There are several risk factors that contribute to the development of VTE. The severity of these risk factors can be measured by quantifying the polarity of sentiments in clinical notes [167] from which the aggregated risk of developing VTE can be determined.

In the context of cardiovascular diseases, sentiment analysis can be used for multiple use cases including monitoring, triage and secondary prevention [22]. In a cardiovascular secondary prevention setting, patients are asked to report their health status on a regular basis by SMS text messaging. These messages can be analysed with sentiment analysis methods for realising the triage and support human monitors [122]. Integrating sentiment analysis into monitoring technologies for disease monitoring of cardiovascular diseases patients supports in precise mining diabetes and heart-related information from social network sites [174]. Sentiment analysis can also help in learning more about risk factors; for example emotional risk factors for cardiovascular diseases can be analysed in social media postings and related to diagnoses, symptoms or outcomes [84].

2.4 Sentiment Analysis for Public Health

Health forums or other social media allow internet users (often non-health professionals) to exchange opinions on their health situation. These platforms are used to express affective states such as emotions, opinions, doubts, risk fears, etc. on treatments, diagnoses or public health interventions. Analysing these resources gives access to interesting information on perception of treatments or personal attitudes. Sentiment analysis has the potential to be a useful tool for public health experts, offering insights into societal attitudes, spotting new health dangers, and enhancing the quality of medical services. There are a number of use cases for sentiment analysis in the field of public health (summarised in Table 2.4). Some examples include:

- Sentiment analysis can be used to track and identify public opinion on a variety of health-related topics, including vaccination reluctance, and public health policy. This can offer insightful information about the attitudes and concerns of the population, which can guide public health campaigns and interventions.
- Sentiment analysis can be used to monitor social media for indications of developing health hazards, such as outbreaks of infectious diseases or food-borne disorders. This will enable public health officials to address these dangers swiftly and successfully.

Table 2.4 Use cases for public health—overview

Information need	Information on population's opinions on public health measures and public health issues, current topics of interest and risks of misinformation
Text sources	Social media
Example use case	Knowledge in population's perceptions and opinions on the current vaccination campaign helps to tune the campaigns's content and strategy. For identified misinformation countermeasures are taken in terms of information campaigns

- Sentiment analysis can be used to spot instances of misinformation, which have a negative effect on behaviour and adherence to public health measures.

Emotion and sentiment analysis of social media content aids in identifying potential flaws in patient education, health information, or other areas where support is needed [1]. It can also help to understand emotions during pandemics. A potential use case during the COVID-19 pandemic was to apply sentiment analysis to understand the population's opinions on health measurements like vaccination campaigns or hygienic measurements as they had been put in place during the pandemic [11]. Samuel et al. applied sentiment analysis to study the Coronavirus fear sentiment progression [169].

Another application area is to study public opinions on public health measures such as birth control [10]. For example, debates on the effects of new generation pills in French forums prompted some women to stop taking contraceptive pills, with a concomitant increase in abortions [24]. By understanding the public sentiment about those topics, government officials and public health policy makers can design more effective communication, education and policy implementation strategies to reach out to the public.

By analysing postings from an online disease community (e.g. Alzheimer's Disease) with respect to sentiment and opinions can help to understand communities' pressing needs [186]. It also helps to get insights into what people know about the disease, or which aspects have a positive or negative impact on them [23]. Knowing the sentiment expressed by social media users towards a disease is important to comprehend what impacts on the people affected with this health condition and their family members [66].

Applying sentiment analysis to patient-written personal statements in the web can uncover trends or underlying patterns. These patterns in turn can help understanding factors involved in clinical outcomes, reasons for non-compliance, as well as analysing patient perceptions and attitudes towards treatments [34] or diseases [66]. For example, web-based parenting forums were analysed regarding topics of concern and sentiments regarding parenting [10]. These examples demonstrate that sentiment analysis has a broad variety of use cases in public health.

2.5 Sentiment Analysis for Pharmacovigilance

Pharmacovigilance is concerned about drug safety and deals with collecting, detecting, assessing, monitoring, and preventing adverse effects with pharmaceutical products. Adverse drug events (ADE) result from drug-related medical events. Many ADE are discovered during drug development in clinical trials that assess the efficacy and side effects of drugs. However, some side effects might not be revealed during this stage due to limited size of clinical trials, the controlled setting and selection of participants [157]. As a result, not all ADE can be identified before a drug is released onto market. Therefore, post-marketing drug surveillance, i.e. pharmacovigilance, plays a major role concerning drug safety once a drug has been released.

Pharmaceutical companies increasingly recognise that online postings can be used to monitor patients' opinions on their products and services, and to obtain feedback on product's performance and consumers' satisfaction [4]. Some of the use cases include (Table 2.5):

- Identifying adverse drug events: Sentiment analysis can be used to analyse patient feedback about medications, such as provided through online reviews. This can assist in locating instances of pharmaceutical side effects, which can help guide pharmacovigilance efforts.
- Monitoring social media for adverse drug events: Sentiment analysis can be used to monitor signals of ADE on social media. This can contribute to the information available for pharmacovigilance efforts and make it easier to recognise potential safety concerns.
- Analysing patient satisfaction with medications: Sentiment analysis can be used to analyse patient feedback about medications to assess patient satisfaction, efficacy in real world application and identify areas for improvement. This can inform pharmacovigilance efforts by providing insights into the effectiveness of medications and the impact they have on patient quality of life [78, 133].

From social media data signals can be retrieved pointing to potential ADE [116, 157]. In particular sentiment analysis can help in identifying judgements of ADE such as negative feelings or a negative opinion on a specific drug [157], but also classifying reported symptoms and perceptions of the personal health under a certain drug treatment. Once a thorough analysis of social media content has been

Table 2.5 Use cases for pharmacovigilance—overview

Information need	Information on adverse events (symptoms), intake behaviour, patient reported outcomes
Text sources	Social media
Example use case	Drug reviews are analysed regarding sentiment and outcomes; Drug reviews are analysed for adverse drug events

conducted, ADE may be logged, and specific preventative actions may be taken to avoid patient harm.

Approaches such as therapy recommender systems, which aim at helping to find an optimal personalised therapy option for a given patient and time, can benefit from feedback on therapy outcomes as retrieved from social media postings on drugs [74]. This requires not only the analysis of expressed sentiment, but also of relevant patient histories.

2.6 Sentiment and Emotion Analysis in Health-Related Conversational Agents

There is an increase of interest in conversational agents integrated in mobile health applications. They allow to interact with a system using natural language and thus simulate the conversation between healthcare professionals and patients. Since this communication is (or should be) characterised by empathy—as patient-doctor communication does—sentiment and emotion analysis becomes relevant for conversational agents in healthcare. Once able to identify the user's emotion and sentiment, the conversational agent can create an empathetic response. The implementation of empathy to interactions with healthcare conversational agents is considered promising since it is a crucial element in doctor-patient relationships [172]. It can even be relevant for deliver an appropriate intervention [51, 52]. The main aim of therapeutic conversational agents for mental health is to understand the appropriate emotions from the user's conversations, suggest appropriate micro-interventions or redirect to a mental health professional in case of any emergencies [54].

Emotion and sentiment in this context comprises subjective, emotional statements that are given by a user while interacting with the conversational agent. Especially while dealing with a mental health patient or even delivering cognitive behavioural therapy (CBT), it is vital to understand the emotional state and respond with simple micro-interventions such as suggestions for a deep breathing exercise or a friendly conversation (Table 2.6). We will outline two examples in the following. CBT shares the idea that behaviour change may be affected via cognitive change. It aims to turn the patient's negative thoughts into positive ones. Within the HABIT project, a mobile application for CBT has been developed that uses a conversational agent for delivery of CBT [197]. An emotion analyser could support in automatically analysing the responses of a user, supporting the therapist in analysing the chatlog afterwards or enabling agent responses that address these moods and tones of user statements. For example a negative answer, high emotional, neglecting a suggestion of the therapist might be interpreted as low acceptance of the immediately prior recommendation. The detected sentiment of a user could also be used to generate motivational suggestions the conversational agent can post to the user targeting at achieving the defined personal health goal.

Table 2.6 Use cases for conversational agents—overview

Information need	Information on the users current emotional state for appropriate reaction
Text sources	Conversations with conversational agents
Example use case	Intelligent agent that suggests micro-interventions to a patient depending on his or her current mood

SERMO is a conversational agent designed for supporting CBT (see Chap. 13), in particular designed for emotion regulation [52]. Based on the free text comments of a user in the chat, the system recognises the current emotion of the user and suggests appropriate measurements and exercises that might help the user in dealing with the emotion in case the user wants to control these emotions. There are similar conversational agents for CBT available that include emotion analysis such as Woebot [61] or Tess [64].

Part II
Resources and Challenges

Chapter 3
Medical Social Media and Its Characteristics

3.1 Characteristics of Medical Social Media Data

Most research on medical sentiment analysis so far considers textual data distributed through social media platforms. Social media refers to online platforms that allow people to connect with each other and share content. Some examples of social media platforms include Facebook, Twitter, Instagram, LinkedIn, and TikTok. The platforms are used to share experiences with treatments or searching for help when getting diagnosed. Individuals connect as patient communities through social media platforms.

Social media platforms typically provide users with a personal profile, a news feed or timeline, and the ability to interact with others through likes, comments, and messages. Users can also create and share their own content, such as text posts, images, and videos. Social media has become an important part of modern life, as it allows people to stay connected with friends and family, access news and information, and participate in online communities. However, it has also raised concerns about privacy, cyberbullying [38], and the spread of misinformation [195].

Social media differs in terms of language from clinical narratives due to the author, purpose and context of writing. Authors of medical social media postings are often individuals who either have a health problem, undergo some treatment or are informal caregivers. Some of the purposes of writing social media postings are: raising discussions, seeking for help, expressing opinions, or describing experiences in living with diseases or with treatments. Given these purposes, authors of social media data write in a rather subjective manner. Compared to language use in clinical narratives, social media texts contain more verbs and adjectives [48]. Also the type of verbs used differs: they are referring to effects of medical procedures, drugs and proteins or genes (e.g. *affect, regulate*), to education and research (e.g. *learn, discuss, study, empower, educate*). The verbs are often used to describe disease development and transfer (e.g. *contribute, depend, infect, require, acquire*). In contrast to clinical narratives, personal pronouns and verbs as well

K. Denecke, *Sentiment Analysis in the Medical Domain*,
https://doi.org/10.1007/978-3-031-30187-2_3

as a variety of adjectives are used. Everyday language is combined with medical terminology. Besides of using medical terminology for describing diseases and medical conditions, layman vocabulary is used [48].

Other linguistic characteristics of medical social media include: use of hashtags, abbreviations, emoticons, linguistic variations of the same concept, informal language, non-standard grammar, and typos. Emoticons are used to convey emotions or give contextual information to correctly understand a message (irony, sarcasm) [50]. Conversations or statements from others can be cited, which aggravates determining the opinion holder. In terms of content, social media postings contain a mixture of facts and experiences or opinions.

In social media, we have to deal with the fact that postings can be in different languages or we are even interested in data from different regions around the world. A challenge here is then to deal with multiple languages. Sentiment analysis approaches are often language-specific, in particular when relying upon trained models or lexical resources.

Besides the availability of some ready-to-use social media datasets—even already annotated with sentiments—web data can be crawled from the web using web crawler or APIs of the social media provider (e.g. Twitter API). Even though easier to retrieve than clinical narratives, current legal regulations and terms of use have to be considered when crawling medical web data. In the following, we list sources that have been exploited within the previously mentioned use cases. We outline the peculiarities of each source including linguistic challenges.

3.2 Twitter

Twitter is a public social media platform with users of vastly different cultural backgrounds and knowledge levels. It has been used for monitoring the dynamics of public opinion and health behaviour during COVID-19 pandemic [21]. It also provides insights into experiences and feelings regarding physical rehabilitation [205]. Tweets allow only for messages of a length of 280 characters and often contain URLs, emojis, special characters, hash symbols, and hyperlinks pointing to websites. Some of this information is irrelevant for sentiment analysis (e.g. URLs); others like emojis are used by their authors to express sentiments. An example is shown in Fig. 3.1.

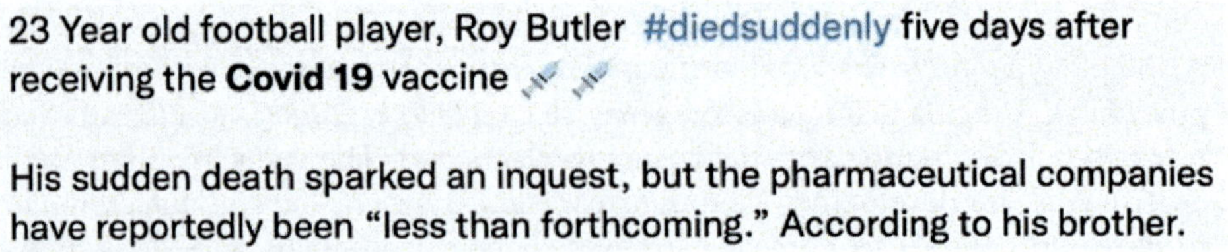
23 Year old football player, Roy Butler #diedsuddenly five days after receiving the **Covid 19** vaccine

His sudden death sparked an inquest, but the pharmaceutical companies have reportedly been "less than forthcoming." According to his brother.

Fig. 3.1 Example tweet

Tweets often use informal language and slang, and may contain unconventional grammar or spelling. This is because tweets are often intended to be conversational and casual, and are not as formal as other forms of written communication. New words can occur, new meanings of already known words can be introduced (e.g. *Bieber-Fever* referring to excitement around Justin Bieber).

The most common features of language on Twitter are slang, new words, abbreviations, emoticons, hashtags (e.g. in the example *#diedsuddenly*) and grammatical errors. Hashtags, which are words or phrases preceded by a "#" symbol, are used to categorise and organise tweets. They allow users to easily search for and find tweets on a particular topic.

Beyond these rather general characteristics of tweets, it can be noted that depending on the community or topic, the characteristics differ. For example, a study demonstrated that suicide-related tweets have unique linguistic profiles [152]. It is recommendable, to analyse the word usage of the community or topic under consideration to adjust the medical sentiment analysis techniques accordingly.

Twitter can be accessed via its API.[1] Some datasets are ready to use for sentiment analysis experiments, even though not specifically collected for medical sentiment analysis. To mention a few of them:

- Sentiment140 (n = 498, https://www.kaggle.com/datasets/kazanova/sentiment140),
- Kaggle (n = 7086, [154]), and
- Sanders dataset (n = 5113, https://github.com/zfz/twitter_corpus#).

are publicly available datasets specifically labelled for sentiment analysis. These datasets contain tweets on any topic, not specifically medical-related ones.

3.3 User Reviews

On review websites, users post reviews or express their opinions about a particular topic (e.g. healthcare service, healthcare provider, drug, medical device etc.). Various sources are available that contain user reviews of drugs [37], of health apps (e.g. customer reviews from Google Play Store [156]), or medical products.

Drugs.com is a provider of pharmaceutical information providing information for both, consumers and healthcare professionals. In addition to information on expected drug use, side effects and common dosage information, it provides user reviews on drugs along with related medical conditions and a 10-star user rating reflecting overall user satisfaction. Figure 3.2 shows the rating overview for the drug Echinacea. Table 3.1 shows two example reviews for this drug.

Similarly, Druglib.com is a resource of drug information for both, consumer and healthcare professionals. Drug reviews contain information related to multiple aspects such as effectiveness of drugs and side effects. Reviews are split into

[1] https://developer.twitter.com/en/docs/twitter-api.

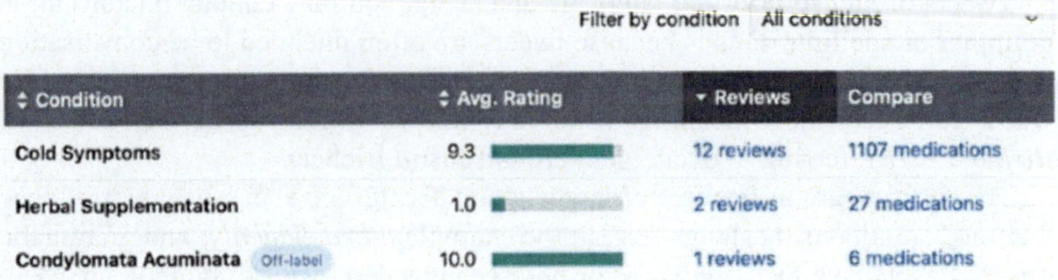

Fig. 3.2 Overview on ratings at Drugs.com on Echinacea. Ratings are grouped according to medical conditions

Table 3.1 Two example reviews from Drugs.com for Echinacea

"I had a upper respiratory infection, including yellow green phlegm and a nasty sore throat from all of the sinus drip. My naturopath prescribed a capsule mix of echinacea and goldenseal that I took 4 times a day for one week, and proof my sinus/respiratory infection was gone. In the past I've always taken antibiotics for these kind of sinus problems that crop up in the winter, but I'm glad to have found a more natural alternative that returns some needed vitamins and nutrients to my body while ridding me of a nasty condition."
"OMG! Totally amazing med. Had a hum dinger of a cold on Friday, came all of a sudden during this now present flu season. I Took pills around clock all day/nite, on Sat. BY SUNDAY MY COLD WAS ALL GONE AND DRAINING ALL FROM NOSE INSTEAD OF CHEST. Not only did it take away my awful cold, I GOT ENERGY FROM WHERE I DO NOT KNOW. THIS MED WAS VERY EFFECTIVE.

three aspects: benefits, side effects and overall comment. Similar to Drugs.com, ratings are available concerning overall satisfaction. Additionally, a 5-step side effect rating, ranging from no side effects to extremely severe side effects and a 5-step effectiveness rating ranging from ineffective to very effective is provided. Both data sources have been used by Graesser et al. [75] for aspect-based sentiment analysis of drug reviews.

Another source of drug reviews are WebMD[2] drug reviews. They provide structured information on drugs in terms of ratings on a 5-point scale and free-textual information. For example, information on the indication for which the drug was consumed is collected, information on the receiver (age, sex, whether the reviewer is the patient himself or someone else), on the effectiveness rated on a scale of 1–5, on the ease of use (user friendliness of the drug on a scale of 1–5), or satisfaction. Finally, a comment can be provided including effects and improvements, i.e. experiences of the patient caused by the consumption of the drug.

Drug reviews may include descriptions of the intended use and effects of a medication, as well as information about side effects, dosage, and potential interactions with other medications. Their authors use technical phrases and medical jargon exclusive to the pharmacology industry. Drug reviews may not just contain technical

[2] http://www.wedmd.com.

jargon but also anecdotes from the reviewer's own life and their perceptions of the treatment, such as how well it worked for them or any side effects they encountered.

The web also provides reviews on healthcare provider, e.g. RateMD or Good Doctor Online. Those reviews directly reflect patients' real opinions on physicians or hospitals, the perceived trustworthiness and can be considered as electronic word of mouth. Liu et al. used online reviews related to a telemedicine service called Online Private Doctor to determine topics patients are talking about related to the telemedicine service and whether they are satisfied with the service or not [120].

The examples show that reviews most often comprise a star-based rating and a freetextual description. The length of a review comment is not restricted and can be quite long. Individuals are describing their experience with the drug or healthcare service. For drug reviews entire histories of illness can be found, comparison to previous medications etc. Linguistically, the spectrum is huge, ranging from complete sentences, to purely subjective statements with exclamations. Sentiments can be strengthened by capitalisation (e.g. "I had TERRIBLE insomnia with this medication.").

3.4 Forums

In forums such as Reddit, people discuss different types of questions, share their thoughts and ideas or provide support by sending messages to questions. Reddit aims at enabling users sharing text-based posts with others. The subforum function (called subreddits) allows creating groups to interact with users over a shared interest. This user-generated content often contains sentiments and emotions, in particular when problems are discussed. Reddit has several subreddits related to health topics such as the subreddit about cancer.[3] In contrast to Twitter, Reddit does not restrict the length of postings, leading to more comprehensive postings. Foufi et al. used Reddit posts to study biomedical entities found in health social media platforms and the way how people suffering from chronic diseases express themselves [63]. The example posting in Table 3.2 shows that the author is mentioning his disease and expressing his thoughts and sentiments.

NHS Choices is a website hosted by the National Health Service (NHS, http://nhs.uk), which provides knowledge on health-related queries. Besides providing articles about various medical conditions and medications, it offers users the option to rate and comment on healthcare services. This user feedback can provide a source for medical sentiment analysis experiments [176]. Patients provide both ratings and reviews for a particular NHS clinic. It was exploited by Bahja et al. for studying patient experiences with healthcare services [7].

[3] https://www.reddit.com/r/cancer/.

Table 3.2 Example post from Reddit

Hi all, I (22M) was just diagnosed with Ewing's sarcoma. I have been through a range of emotions and I'm trying so hard to put on a brave face, but this is really starting to weigh on me. Usually when I'm having a hard time I retreat from everyone, which kind of makes me more sad but people usually know me as the energetic, always on, always engaging, entertaining guy. I want to show everyone that I'm not scared, but I can feel this increasingly weighing on my mind as I prepare to start chemo on Wednesday. I'm in my last semester of college and I feel less motivated than ever. I feel like whenever I try to visualise my future, it's extremely opaque and that really kills me. Is there anyone else around this age (or dealt with cancer at this age) who has any advice/encouragement? I'm having such a hard time shaking this feeling

The MedHelp[4] health site provides the opportunity to form communities and share information and opinions about diseases. Each community consists of a number of conversations; a conversation being a sequence of comments posted by patients. Postings of this forum have been aggregated in a dataset and annotated with sentiments (see Chap. 6). Content-wise forum texts are longer texts with personal anecdotes and descriptions. They can reflect knowledge on diseases or treatments. Forums are often used to seek help; thus, postings may contain questions. Forum postings can have a wide range of linguistic characteristics, as they are written by people from diverse backgrounds and with different writing styles and educational levels. Some common characteristics of forum postings include the use of colloquial language, abbreviations, emoticons, and nonstandard grammar and spelling. Similarly to tweets or review texts, forum postings may also contain slang, jargon, and technical terms, depending on the topic being discussed. Given their length, forum postings may include elements of humour, irony, and sarcasm. It is important to keep in mind that their linguistic characteristics can vary widely depending on the authors, and generalisations are often difficult.

[4] http://www.medhelp.org/.

Chapter 4
Clinical Narratives and Their Characteristics

4.1 Linguistic Characteristics of Clinical Narratives

Clinical narratives are written in a rather descriptive, objective manner instead of an opinionated manner (e.g. a sentence like *the patient presented with headaches*). The purpose of clinical documentation differs from the purpose of medical social media. Clinical documentation is legally required to document the treatment process for reimbursement purposes. Opinions are not explicitly formulated, but rather subtle or even captured in the word semantics. This leads to a rather low number of sentiment terms used in clinical texts (5–10% in clinical narratives [49]). Observations of a health professional regarding the patient's health status, but also on physical appearances are aspects that can be found described in a rather objective manner.

Uncertainty is explicitly stated and typical for clinical narratives. For example a phrase like *Suspicion of diabetes* could be part of one of the first documentations within a treatment process. The clinical diagnosing process often starts from assumptions and examinations conducted to confirm or reject these assumptions. In addition to the mentioned characteristics, the language used in clinical narratives is formal and often contains medical terminology to a large extent which is unique for these text types. Indirect speech can be used which complicates the identification of the opinion holder (e.g. in the sentence "Patient's spouse reports some episodes of dysphagia." which originates from a nurse report). Consequently, applying state of the art tools designed for general purpose sentiment analysis to clinical narratives has not been proven to be successful [49].

4.2 Clinical Narratives

Clinical narratives are normally considered to be collections of facts summarising the medical condition and treatment of a patient. They must be accurate, timely

K. Denecke, *Sentiment Analysis in the Medical Domain*,
https://doi.org/10.1007/978-3-031-30187-2_4

and reflect specific healthcare services provided to a patient. Some types of clinical narratives refer to supporting electronic files such as magnetic resonance imaging (MRI) scans, X-rays, electrocardiograms (ECG) or records of monitoring. They are used to facilitate inter-provider communication and provide evidence for legal records. Written in an objective manner one might ask where we can find medical sentiment in such documents. Besides summarising the treatment, they mainly reflect the observations of physicians and health carers and their interpretation of medical data. Consider diagnoses: depending on the phase of the medical decision making process, a diagnosis might be preliminary, a suspicion. Severity of symptoms is also a subjective aspect. During the patient contact, physicians collect and reflect on the patient's quality of life—again a subjective judgement. In summary, clinical narratives normally summarise objectively the health status of a patient, diagnosis and procedures. Personal judgements of a physician concern the patient's health status change, e.g. *the patient recovered well* and interpretations of factual data like medical images [48].

The process and outcomes of in-hospital care of patients is documented in several documents including admission notes, radiology reports, progress notes, discharge summaries or nursing notes. Clinical narratives summarise clinical manifestations and treatment processes. Beyond, they contain the observations of health professionals regarding a patient's health. They describe information on diagnosis, medications, complications occurred during a treatment, on findings etc. Beyond, biochemical information (e.g. gas exchange in the lungs), functional information (e.g. blood flow in vessels) or morphological information (e.g. CT scan) is often part of clinical data.

An admission note documents a patient's status, reasons of admission and the initial instructions for follow-up patient care. Hospital admission notes include the personal information of the patient, the medical examination report, accommodation and relative's information among other important information about the patient's status.

Nursing or progress notes bear valuable information on the health status of a patient. They are typically characterised by the use of specific terminology related to nursing care and patient assessment. They include descriptions of the patient's physical condition, including vital signs, symptoms, and any treatments or interventions that have been administered. In addition, nursing notes may also include observations about the patient's behaviour, mood or on the psychological status [86], and overall functioning, as well as recommendations for further care or treatment.

A radiology report describes observations in radiological images including X-rays, CT scans, and MRIs, the corresponding finding, anomalies seen and their interpretation. The use of technical jargon and specialised terminology linked to medical imaging and the interpretation of diagnostic pictures is a common feature of radiology reports. They may contain technical terminology in addition to details on a patient's medical history. They may also contain suggestions for future testing or follow-up therapy.

A discharge summary is written at the end of a treatment process and summarises the hospital stay of a patient (which procedures were taken, which diagnoses have been assured, which medications have been prescribed). Discharge summaries may include descriptions of the patient's medical history, diagnosis, and treatment while in the hospital, as well as any follow-up care or treatment that is recommended after the patient has been discharged. These descriptions may include medical terms and technical language that is specific to the field of medicine.

Since they are part of the clinical documentation, these are legal documents required for legal or billing purposes or for communication purposes (e.g. for information exchange between physicians). Even though they are containing observations and subjective judgements they are written in a neutral manner often without explicitly using sentiment-bearing terms. Personal impressions expressed in clinical narratives concern perceptions of a health carer towards a patient's health status (e.g. the phrase patient recovered well) and interpretations of medical images and examination results.

Chapter 5
Other Data Sources

5.1 User Statements from Interaction with Intelligent Agents

Intelligent agents are increasingly used to mimic human conversation. In this way, they are starting to change not only how businesses interact with their customers, but also how healthcare professionals interact with patients and how health interventions are delivered to the patient.

User interaction with intelligent agents with conversational user interface leads to user statements that may contain expressions of sentiments. Depending on the system's scope and interaction possibilities, these user statements can be more or less comprehensive. Integrating sentiment or emotion analysis in health-related conversational agents requires analysis of user input phrases from the interaction with the agent [52]. I.e. conversation statements are an additional data source for medical sentiment analysis.

Conversational sentiment is more nuanced than that found in movie or customer reviews. All the information needed to determine sentiment in a piece of text is contained in a movie or product review. In contrast, the user's reaction in a conversation with an intelligent agent depends on what the agent is saying and in what context. The expressed opinion can be spread over several conversation turns. In contrast to a review, a conversation's tone is always shifting as each participant speaks. Therefore, determining the sentiment of a conversation requires taking into account both what each speaker is saying and dynamic changes brought on by each speaker's contributions, be it the agent or the user.

K. Denecke, *Sentiment Analysis in the Medical Domain*,
https://doi.org/10.1007/978-3-031-30187-2_5

5.2 Other Sources

Another source for applying sentiment analysis in the medical domain are PubMed abstracts. PubMed[1] is a bibliographic database of biomedical literature. It contains more than 34 million citations and abstracts of biomedical literature. Data entries normally comprise metadata such as author names, title of the publication, journal, publication type etc. and the abstract. A few full texts are available directly, but often a link to the publisher is provided to access the full text. Biomedical literature (e.g. paper on clinical trials) has been analysed using sentiment analysis with respect to the outcome of a medical treatment [151]. Sentiment analysis was also applied to PubMed abstracts to classify the importance or potential impact of the reported results [60].

The linguistic characteristics of the articles (or abstracts) in PubMed depends on the language in which the article was written and the subject matter being discussed. In general, the language used in scientific articles is more formal and technical than the language used in social media. Scientific writing tends to use precise, specific language and follows a standard structure that includes an introduction, methods, results, and discussion section. Scientific articles may also include technical terms and jargon specific to the field of study, as well as citations to other research. The language used in scientific articles is designed to be clear and concise, and to convey information in a way that is easily understood by other researchers in the field.

Additional sources of data for medical sentiment analysis are free-text answers to open-ended questions in PROM questionnaires [181], online questionnaires with open ended questions [124] or feedback systems for patients. The most valuable and direct feedback are patient complaints. Patient complaints can help healthcare organisations identify unsafe and dissatisfying behaviours as well as avoidable variability in performance. Reported observations of patients and families to healthcare organisations in the form of spontaneous complaints of unprofessional behaviour have been used for analysing sentiment by Messiry et al. [57]. Their complaints were retrieved from the Patient Advocacy Reporting System (PARS). PARS was developed at Vanderbilt Center for Patient and Professional Advocacy. It is used at more than 140 other medical centers to capture, classify, and address such complaints [85].

[1] https://pubmed.ncbi.nlm.nih.gov.

Chapter 6
Datasets for Medical Sentiment Analysis

6.1 The Burden of Available Datasets

One major challenge for medical sentiment analysis is the lack of annotated data. Especially, labelled data dealing with distinct aspects is rare [75]. Moreover, the availability of labelled data is highly domain dependent. For some diseases, more data is available than for others (e.g. many postings from persons with diabetes are available while for other diseases data is rare). Availability of a sufficient amount of data is crucial for accurate sentiment classification, in particular when relying upon supervised machine learning. Even larger data sets are needed for deep learning techniques to learn, for instance, embeddings. Since clinical data is rare, a solution in latter case is to enrich embedding vectors trained for example on Wikipedia data or other freely available data with a smaller amount of domain-specific data.

Assembling a medical social media dataset goes along with additional difficulties: Only certain subsets of the enormous amounts of social media data that might be gathered may be pertinent for a particular use case needing medical sentiment analysis. For instance, a dataset comprising postings related to a specific (health) topic are of relevance, i.e. mentioning specific terms or written by a particular user group (e.g. tweets from autistic people). Noise and spam can be contained within the collection of tweets or other social media postings, but they must be recognised before processing in order to prevent the medical sentiment analysis results from being of poor quality. Therefore, before using sentiment analysis, it is essential to reduce the amount of noise or spam (remove adverts and announcements from news agencies).

K. Denecke, *Sentiment Analysis in the Medical Domain*,
https://doi.org/10.1007/978-3-031-30187-2_6

6.2 MIMIC Databases

The MIMIC Corpus (Medical Information Mart for Intensive Care) comprises data from hospital admissions requiring ICU care at the Beth Israel Deaconess Medical Center in Boston, Massachusetts, between 2001 and 2012 [99]. It is continuously updated with more recent clinical data. While the original database only contained data from patients at ICUs, the most recent databases include data from emergency departments [101].

Data within the MIMIC databases includes vital signs and physiologic signals, medications, laboratory measurements, observations and notes charted by care providers, fluid balance, procedure codes, diagnostic codes, imaging reports, hospital length of stay, survival data, and more for tens of thousands of Intensive Care Unit (ICU) patients. The MIMIC II Clinical Database contains clinical data from bedside workstations as well as hospital archives. It contains data collected between 2001 and 2008 from a variety of ICUs (medical, surgical, coronary care, and neonatal).

The MIMIC III database comprises additional MIMIC II data and additional data until 2012, in total for over 40,000 patients. The MIMIC-III database is now accessible on Google Cloud Platform (GCP) and Amazon Web Services, two of the most popular cloud computing platforms (AWS). MIMIC-IV is sourced from two in-hospital database systems: a custom hospital-wide EHR and an ICU-specific clinical information system. The MIMIC Chest X-ray (MIMIC-CXR) Database v2.0.0 is a large publicly available dataset of chest radiographs in DICOM format with free-text radiology reports [100]. Information on all available datasets is provided by PhysioNet.[1]

In particular the nurse letters contained in MIMIC-II and MIMIC-III have been used in the context of medical sentiment analysis. A few examples are listed in the following. Sanglerdsinlapachai et al. used discharge summaries (2504 sentences) from MIMIC-II [170]. Each sentence was annotated with polarity information (positive, negative) resulting in 1237 positive and 1267 negative sentences. Zou et al. applied an out-of-the box sentiment analysis tool (TextBlob) on nursing notes of 1844 sepsis cases retrieved from the MIMIC-III database for predicting the 30-day mortality [210]. Dang et al. manually labelled 6000 sentences of MIMIC-II with two labels: "1" (positive) and "−1" (negative) [41]. Ghassemi et al. used MIMIC III and applied medical sentiment analysis to visualise the evolution of clinical language and sentiment with respect to several common population-level categories including: time in the hospital, age, mortality, gender and race [70]. Using a lexicon match they replaced all positive sentiment terms in the text with the single term 'POSITIVE', and all negative sentiment terms with the single term 'NEGATIVE'. Further, a sentiment score was determined by calculating the ratio of positive to

[1] https://physionet.org/.

negative sentiment expressions in the text. For realising the lexicon match, the collection of negative and positive terms from Liu et al. was used as lexicon [118].

6.3 i2B2 Dataset

A de-identified set of clinical records was provided by the i2B2 initiative (Informatics for Integrating Biology and the Bedside) for several natural language processing challenges. The tasks and data previously conducted through i2b2 are now are housed in the Department of Biomedical Informatics at Harvard Medical School as n2c2: National NLP Clinical Challenges.[2] Challenges have been conducted since 2006 addressing different tasks. For these challenges, datasets with different clinical scopes have been generated (e.g. obesity, medication, heart disease, psychiatry). Each dataset is annotated with task-specific data which is—except for one dataset—not related to medical sentiment. The goal of the 2009 i2b2 NLP challenge was for example to extract medication information from de-identified hospital discharge summaries, including medication name, dosage, mode, frequency, duration, and cause.

The Obesity Challenge data consists of 1237 discharge summaries. The data were taken from the discharge summaries of patients who had been hospitalised since December 1, 2004, for either obesity- or diabetes-related reasons, and who were overweight or diabetic [193]. It was used for medical sentiment analysis by Chen et al. [32].

The I2B2/VA/Cincinnati 2011 Natural Language Processing (NLP) Challenge had a track on sentiment classification in suicide notes. The data originated from a collection of over 1000 notes that were written by people who had committed suicide. The data are hand annotated with emotions [159]. More specifically, 15 emotions had to be distinguished at the sentence-level within these suicide notes. Six hundred suicide notes were provided as training material [179].

Another challenge was the i2b2 heart failure challenge. The dataset comprises 1304 de-identified longitudinal medical records describing 296 patients, selected to support research into the progression of Coronary Artery Disease (CAD) in diabetic patients. This data was used for determining the risk of heart failure disease using sentiment analysis [184].

6.4 TREC Dataset

The Text REtrieval Conference (TREC) runs information retrieval challenges and includes a medical track series (http://trec-cds.org, [33]). These tracks have sought

[2] https://n2c2.dbmi.hms.harvard.edu/.

to provide benchmark datasets and evaluate information retrieval systems focused on many of the most important information access problems in biomedicine. One track focused on retrieving cohorts of patients from electronic health records. The provided dataset comprises biomedical documents and clinical narratives from PubMed. This dataset was used by Sabra et al. for prediction of venous thromboembolism using sentiment analysis [167].

6.5 eDiseases Dataset

The eDiseases dataset is a social media dataset [28]. It contains patient data from the MedHelp health site (http://www.medhelp.org/). To build the dataset, ten conversations from three communities: allergies, crohn and breast cancer were retrieved. The conversations were selected randomly, filtering out conversations with less than 10 posts. In total, the dataset comprises 146 posts (983 sentences) on allergies, 191 posts (1780 sentences) on crohn, and 142 posts (1029 sentences) on breast cancer covering a 6-years time interval. Three frequent users of health forums annotated each sentence in the dataset with factuality (three possible values: opinion, fact, experience) and polarity (positive, neutral, negative).

6.6 Multimodal Sentiment Analysis Challenge (MuSe)

MuSe is a competition aimed at comparing multimedia processing and deep learning methods for automatic, integrated audiovisual, and textual based sentiment and emotion sensing, under a common experimental condition set. In the 2022 competitions there are two challenges related to emotion analysis:

1. The Emotional Reactions Sub-Challenge aimed at predicting the intensities of emotions. The focus was on seven self-reported emotions that had to be extracted from user-generated reactions to emotionally evocative videos. The sub-challenge was based on the Hume-React data set (see below).
2. The Multimodal Emotional Stress Sub-challenge (MuSe-Stress) aimed at predicting the level of valence and psycho-physiological arousal in a time-continuous manner from audio-visual recordings. It was based on the Ulm-TSST database (see below) featuring people in a stressed disposition.

The datasets are multimodal, i.e. comprise not only textual data, but other data types. Hume-React includes about 75 hours of user-generated content. The recordings show a user's reaction to an emotional stimulus. The videos are labelled for seven fine-grained emotions: adoration, amusement, anxiety, disgust, empathic pain, fear and surprise. The Ulm-TSST database[3] contains a multimodal annotated dataset of self-reported, and external dimensional ratings of emotion and mental well-being. It includes biological recordings, such as Electrocardiogram (ECG), Electrodermal Activity (EDA), Respiration, and Heart Rate (BPM) as well as continuous arousal and valence annotations.

6.7 General Domain Datasets

Several social media datasets are available without specific focus on medical content. The *Sentiment-140 dataset* contains 1600000 tweets in English extracted using the Twitter API [72]. The tweets have been annotated (0 = negative, 2 = neutral, 4 = positive). Additionally, a test set of 177 negative tweets and 182 positive tweets with only some data containing emoticons is provided. The training data was post-processed. Emoticons were removed for training purposes. Re-tweets or tweets copied from another user have been removed. The Sentiment-140 dataset was used to train a LSTM model for sentiment classification in the context of depression detection to analyse user input to a web platform [140]. The data is available through Kaggle[4] and other platforms.

A dataset on *global reactions related to COVID-19 on Twitter* has been provided by Gupta et al. [81]. This large dataset reflects the public conversation on Twitter surrounding the COVID-19 pandemic. Each public tweet was annotated with seventeen latent semantic attributes using natural language processing techniques and machine-learning based algorithms. The latent semantic attributes include: (1) ten attributes indicating the tweet's relevance to ten detected topics, (2) five quantitative attributes indicating the degree of intensity in the valence (i.e., unpleasantness/pleasantness) and emotional intensities across four primary emotions of fear, anger, sadness and joy, and (3) two qualitative attributes indicating the sentiment category and the most dominant emotion category, respectively.

The *Stanford Sentiment Treebank SST-2 dataset* is a corpus of movie reviews with fully labelled parse trees [178]. Given these annotations, it allows to fully analyse how sentiment affects language's composition. It contains 215154 phrases with fine-grained sentiment labels in the parse trees of 11855 sentences.

The *Emotional Tweets* dataset contains tweets annotated with six classes. Two classes, joy and surprise, express positive emotions, whereas the others (sadness, fear, anger, disgust) reflect negative emotions. The dataset comprises 21051 labelled tweets [137]. It was used by Imran et al. for training their emotion classifier for analysing reactions and sentiments of citizens from different cultures related to the Coronavirus [95].

---

3 https://www.muse-challenge.org/challenge/data.

4 https://www.kaggle.com/datasets/kazanova/sentiment140.

There are some conversation datasets available annotated with emotions and sentiment, but from the general domain:

DailyDialog[5] is a human-written multi-turn dialog data set that represents daily communication. The data is manually labelled with communication intention and emotional information. It contains 13118 multi-turn dialogues [110].

ScenarioSA is a manually labelled dataset collected from various websites that provide online communication services [207]. The 2214 multi-speaker English conversations are labelled with sentiment labels at sentence-level. Additionally, the sentiment at the end of the conversation is annotated for each speaker [208].

[5] http://yanran.li/dailydialog.html.

Chapter 7
Lexical Resources for Medical Sentiment Analysis

7.1 LIWC

Several lexical resources exist for medical sentiment analysis (Table 7.1). Linguistic Inquiry and Word Counts (LIWC) is a tool for automated text analysis. It calculates the degree to which various categories of words are used in text. Its original purpose is to support psychological research with language data. It helps in revealing people's thoughts, feelings, personality, and sentiments based on a given text written by an individual [189].

LIWC-22 comes with over 100 dictionaries created to capture people's social and psychological states. Each dictionary consists of a list of words, word stems, emoticons, and other specific verbal constructions that have been identified to reflect a psychological category of interest.[1] The word categories correspond to different psychometric properties, for example, different affect processes including positive and negative emotions, like anger, and anxiety.

For instance, the dictionary on "cognitive processes" includes more than 1000 entries that reflect when a person is actively processing information. It comprises for example the cognitive processes of insight (e.g. think, know), causation or inhibition. The "affiliation" dictionary includes over 350 entries that reflect a person's need to connect with others, including words like "community" and "together".

Many LIWC-22 categories are organised in a hierarchical structure. This means for example that all anger words are categorised as negative emotion words, which are in turn categorised as emotion words. Additionally, the same word may be categorised in multiple dictionaries. For instance, the word "celebrate" is contained in both, the dictionary with the positive emotions and the "achievement" dictionary (examples from the liwc.app Website).

[1] https://www.liwc.app/help/howitworks.

K. Denecke, *Sentiment Analysis in the Medical Domain*,
https://doi.org/10.1007/978-3-031-30187-2_7

Table 7.1 Sentiment lexicons

Lexicon name	Sentiment/emotion categories	Task that can be supported	Example
LIWC	Positive, negative	LIWC can be used to identify sentiment in text as well as to gain insights into how people are feeling or thinking when they write or speak	[121, 128]
SentiWordNet	Polarity scores; A triple of values between 0 and 1 reflecting neutrality, positivity and negativity	Sentiment analysis	[70, 117]
SentiHealth	Positive, negative, neutral	Sentiment analysis	[166]
AFINN	Positive, negative (integer ranging from minus 5 to plus 5	Sentiment analysis	[12, 199]
EmoLex	Joy, sadness, anger, fear, trust, disgust, surprise and anticipation, positive, negative	Emotion analysis	[199]
WordNet Affect	Positive, negative, neutral, ambiguous and 28 subcategories (e.g. joy, love, fear)	Sentiment analysis, emotion detection	[180]
WordNet for Medical Events	Polarity score, sentiment (positive, negative, neutral), affinity score, gravity score	Sentiment analysis	[143]

LIWC is available in multiple languages including Brazilian, Portuguese, Chinese (Simplified), Chinese (Simplified, v1.5), Chinese (Traditional), Chinese (Traditional, v1.5), Dutch, French, German, Italian, Japanese, Norwegian, Romanian, Russian, Serbian, Spanish, Turkish, and Ukrainian.[2] It was exploited for analysing text messages in correlation to self-reported depression symptom severity [121]. McDonnell et al. compared sensitivity of different versions of LIWC for identifying emotional expression of cancer survivors [128].

7.2 SentiWordNet and Its Derivations

SentiWordNet[3] is a general purpose sentiment lexicon. It is one of the largest lexicons available in this domain. It comprises more than 60000 synsets obtained from WordNet. WordNet is a lexical database of semantic relations between words which links words into semantic relations including synonyms, hyponyms, and meronyms. Within SentiWordNet to each word, three values between 0 and 1

[2] https://www.liwc.app/dictionaries.

[3] https://github.com/aesuli/SentiWordNet.

reflecting the term's positivity, negativity and neutrality is assigned. All three values sum up to 1. SentiWordNet also uses Part of Speech (POS) tagging to distinguish between different forms of words. It is freely distributed for noncommercial use, and licenses are available for commercial applications. The current version SentiWordNet 3.0 is based upon WordNet 3.0 [6]. As WordNet, also SentiWordNet contains only terms in English, but it has been tested in a multilingual context using machine translation [47].

SentiWordNet has also been adapted or transferred to the medical domain. One approach applied word embedding techniques to the original SentiWordNet lexicon. This is to develop an enhanced sentiment lexicon for the medical domain with position encoding as a vector representation method in order to achieve better sentiment classification performance [117]. It has been exploited to analyse ICU provider sentiment [70].

Another approach was used to develop SentiHealth [5]. SentiHealth comprises 1520 words (40% positive, 45% negative and 15% neutral). The sentiment scoring was determined using the scores from SentiWordNet and a domain-specific strategy for assigning scores to the terms in the lexicon. More specifically, bootstrapping was applied to acquire a set of opinion words from manually compiled seed lists of medical terms. SentiHealth was used for detecting mood of cancer patients in online social networks [166].

7.3 AFINN

AFINN is a lexicon of English words rated for valence with an integer between minus five (negative) and plus five (positive) [150]. The version of 2011 comprises 2477 words and phrases manually annotated with an integer between −5 and +5. For example, an entry assigns to the term *accident* the value of "−2". The list was generated using phrases from multiple sources including Twitter. Since its original development, translations have been made available in Finnish, French, Turkish, Polish for download at GitHub.[4] AFINN was used in the context of medical sentiment analysis for example by Weissman et al. who tested various out-of-the-box tools and methods for general domain sentiment analysis for medical purposes [199]. It was also used for identifying loneliness among mental health patients from clinical notes [12].

7.4 EmoLex

EmoLex [138] (also known as NRC Word-Emotion Association Lexicon) is an English term-emotion lexicon. Terms and phrases (unigrams, bigrams) have been

[4] https://github.com/fnielsen/afinn.

manually annotated through Amazon's Mechanical Turk service. The lexicon focuses on eight emotions: joy, sadness, anger, fear, trust, disgust, surprise and anticipation and two sentiments (positive, negative). EmoLex integrates terms from other lexicons such as General Inquirer and WordNet Affect Lexicon. The other selected terms originate from a Google n-gram dataset. The 200 most frequent n-grams per part of speech have been selected. The current version of the lexicon includes 14182 unigrams with associated categories. EmoLex was used for analysing encounter notes of patients with critical illness [199]. Since 2022, the lexicon is available 108 languages created using automatic translation.

7.5 WordNet Affect

The WordNet Affect Lexicon is an extension of WordNet [182]. It includes a subset of synsets representing affective concepts correlated with affective words. I.e. it is a collection of emotion-related words (nouns, verbs, adjectives, and adverbs), classified manually as "positive", "negative", "neutral", or "ambiguous" and categorised into 28 subcategories ("joy", "love", "fear", etc.). WordNet Affect contains 2874 synsets and 4787 words. It has been used by Spasic et al. to analyse suicide notes [180].

7.6 WordNet for Medical Events

WordNet for Medical Events (WME) is a resource comprising medical concepts together with their linguistic and semantic features [142, 144]. The resource was iteratively developed from version WME 1.0 [142] to WME 3.0 [144].

WME provides information on the parts of speeches, glosses, affinity scores, sentiment score and polarity, but also similar sentiment words. Affinity scores range from 0 to 1 and suggest a sentiment linking between medical concepts and their similar sentiment words, with a chance of 1 implying a strong relation. Additionally, the gravity score acknowledges the emotional connection between concepts and their glosses. The gravity score can be a value between -1 and 1, including 0. While -1 denotes a lack of relationship, 0 denotes situations in which a concept or gloss is neutral and has no assigned sentiment. 1 denotes a strong relationship, either positive or negative, helping to determine the proper gloss for an idea.

The initial version of WME 1.0 was prepared from the datasets of the SemEval-2015 Task-65 [142]. The conventional WordNet and an English medical dictionary were additionally used. From the SemEval 2015 Task-6 datasets, 2479 medical events along with their attributes were extracted. By means of an English medical dictionary, the parts of speeches and word-related glosses of medical concepts were retrieved. Additionally, information on semantics, affinity synonyms and hyponyms were collected from WordNet. Polarity and its related sense features of terms were introduced using the sentiment lexicons (e.g. SentiWordNet, SenticNet, Bing Liu's subjectivity list).

For extending the lexicon, additional sources were used such as WordNet and MedicineNet. WME 3.0 contains 10,186 concepts and their assigned semantic and linguistic features as well as categories (diseases, drugs, symptoms, human anatomy).

WME allows for the extraction of relative sense-based words for medical concepts from various knowledge sources and the classification of medical terms into the proper categories (e.g. treatment, disease, etc.). Using the affinity feature, a medical semantic network of concepts can be built to visualise the relationships between concepts.

WME 3.0 was used by Mondal et al. to develop an automated extraction system for identifying medical and non-medical concepts [141]. The polarity scores and sentiments are used as part of the feature set. Another work used WME as domain-based knowledge lexicon coupled with a machine learning approach to extract semantic relations [143]. The approach makes use of the categories and sentiment of the medical concepts retrieved from the lexical resource.

7.7 Other Sentiment Lexicons

There are several efforts related to the generation of sentiment lexicons worth to be mentioned. Not all of the lexicons listed below have been specifically developed for medical purposes. But they have been applied for medical sentiment analysis.

Goeuriot et at. [73] created a domain-specific sentiment lexicon using a corpus of drug reviews and statistical information. The lexicon contains 1446 terms (73% positive, 27% negative).

The Macquarie Semantic Orientation Lexicon (MSOL) contains more than 70000 expressions that explicitly convey positive or negative meaning [139]. It contains around 30458 positive expressions and 45942 negative expressions. The expressions are individual words or multi-word expressions. MSOL is used by Spasic et al. to classify topics and emotions in suicide notes [180].

Bing Liu maintains and freely distributes a sentiment lexicon consisting of lists of strings.[5] It consists of 2006 positive words and 4783 negative words. An interesting aspect of this lexicon is that it includes misspellings, morphological variants, slang, and social media mark-up.

Chopan et al. use hedonometrics to analyse perceptions on plastic surgery in social media [34]. Hedonometrics, a quantitative sentiment analysis procedure, uses

[5] https://www.cs.uic.edu/~liub/FBS/sentiment-analysis.html.

labMT, a word-happiness data set with over 10000 words, to calculate the average happiness score among different subsets of written text (i.e., tweets) [56].

7.8 Ontologies and Biomedical Vocabularies

Several ontologies and biomedical vocabularies exist that can support medical sentiment analysis in different ways. Such vocabularies can be used in the context of medical sentiment analysis for realising health mention analysis (i.e. for entity or topic recognition), for resolving abbreviations or for selecting texts bearing medical content.

The multilingual, international standard system of clinical terms, SNOMED CT, was created in 2002 and constitutes a medical terminology organised as a directed graph with concepts as nodes and relationships as edges. The core components in SNOMED CT are concepts, descriptions and relationships. A concept represents a unique clinical meaning, which is referenced using a unique, numeric and machine-readable SNOMED CT identifier (e.g. C0038351 for stomach). It consists of more than 350000 concepts and 1000000 relationships that connect concepts. SNOMED CT offers a semantic resource which provides a standardised way to represent phrases describing medical content. Concepts within SNOMED CT cover multiple medical categories: clinical findings, body structure, procedures, social context, substance, physical objects, organisms, pharmaceutical/biological products etc.

Carchiolo et al. monitored health related information using both Twitter data and medical terms present in the SNOMED CT terminology [27], i.e. SNOMED CT is used for identifying tweets dealing with medical issues. Work still has to be done to more deeply explore SNOMED CT and its use for medical sentiment analysis, for instance by exploiting relationships between concepts for a more effective health-related tweets extraction.

The Unified Medical Language System (UMLS) integrates and distributes key terminology, classification systems and coding standards, and associated resources of the medical domain [20]. It consists of three main components: the Metathesaurus, the Semantic Network and the Specialist Lexicon & Lexical Tools. The Metathesaurus is a database of over one million biomedical concepts from 100 different source vocabularies including ICD-10 and SNOMED CT. The Metathesaurus consists of concepts and relations. A single concept can be expressed by many terms. Similar to SNOMED CT, these terms are organised in the UMLS into concepts and a single term is selected as a "preferred term" which is used as a representative of the concept. Several properties are attached to a concept such as source, unique identifier and definition. To each concept in the Metathesaurus at least one semantic type is assigned (see below). Relations connect concepts to each other. Each relation has properties such as source or type.

Kumar et al. are using the UMLS within their sentiment analysis framework to expand acronyms and abbreviations [107]. Niu et al. [151] exploit the UMLS together with the mapping tool MetaMap to identify semantic categories which are used as features in their sentiment analysis algorithm. MetaMap is used to map the text to UMLS concepts. Afterwards, for each concept the semantic category is retrieved from the UMLS and used as feature. Smith et al. extracted the target of the sentiment using MetaMap [176].

Part III
Solutions

Chapter 8
Levels and Tasks of Sentiment Analysis

8.1 Level of Analysis

Sentiment can be studied at several levels: Document-level, sentence-level, and aspect-level (see Fig. 8.1). The aspect-level is the most fine-grained level of analysis, and also the most challenging. Which level to choose depends on the objective of the analysis and the problem under consideration. For some use cases, document-level analysis is sufficient—for others not. Depending on the level of analysis, the linguistic peculiarities become more relevant to be addressed for achieving good sentiment analysis results—or they can be ignored. For example analysing coordination structures is redundant when analysing the sentiment on a document-level since the polarity of all terms of a document will be aggregated (except for negations whose interpretation requires a more detailed assessment). More details on the different levels are described in the following.

8.1.1 Document-Level Sentiment Analysis

Document-level sentiment analysis aims at finding a sentiment polarity for an entire document. The document is expected to have one main topic towards which the opinion holder is expressing the sentiment. For example, when analysing the sentiment of a nurse letter, the opinion of the nurse who wrote the letter towards a specific patient's health status is determined assuming that the nurse letter deals with the patient‘s health status. For a document that compares or describes two or more entities or topics, a document-level sentiment analysis is unsuited since it won't be possible to know for which entity the sentiment holds true. Another challenge of document-level sentiment analysis is that contrasting polarities can compensate each other due to an aggregation at document-level. Consider the example in Fig. 8.2: The entire drug review is classified as negative since the

K. Denecke, *Sentiment Analysis in the Medical Domain*,
https://doi.org/10.1007/978-3-031-30187-2_8

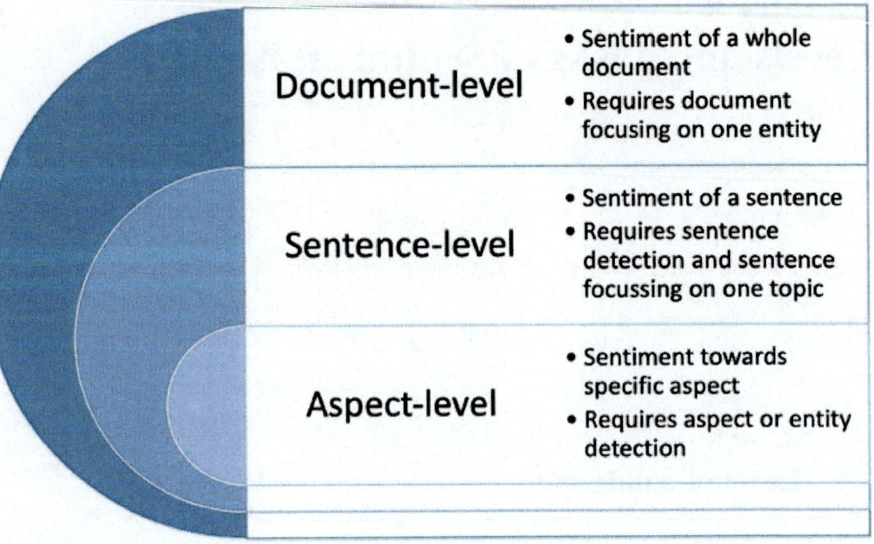

Fig. 8.1 The three levels of sentiment analysis and their requirements

aggregation of the single sentiments allows for this conclusion. Three sentences have been detected as negative; one as positive; one as neutral. At document-level, we are loosing the information on the sentiment of individual sentences. However, in many cases, document-level sentiment analysis can already provide interesting information. Bahja et al. applied a document-level sentiment analysis approach to classify patient feedback posted at the social media platform NHS Choices as positive or negative [7].

8.1.2 Sentence-Level Sentiment Analysis

Sentence-level sentiment analysis first identifies sentences in a document and then classifies them according to sentiment (e.g. positive, negative, neutral or other sentiment categories) [87]. A preceding step of the actual sentence-level sentiment detection is the classification of a sentence as sentiment-bearing or not sentiment-bearing (see subjectivity analysis in Sect. 8.2.1). Assuming that only subjective sentences express a sentiment, this processing step can reduce the number of sentences to be analysed in the following processing steps.

Being more fine grained than document-level sentiment analysis, sentence-level sentiment analysis can capture changes of sentiment across the sentences of a document (see example in Fig. 8.2). But still, it does not provide details on the sentiment regarding specific aspects or medical entities that are expressed in a document. Consider a sentence combining two aspects such as *"Drinking behaviour*

This drug is absolutely helpful for chest pain. Last time I'm agonizing because I didn't warm up for swimming activity. I took mefenamic acid and it didn't work at all. I can't sleep because of pain in my left chest and back. I took 40 mg of Aspilet/Aspirin and after few hours, I got relived!

This document is: negative (-0.56)

Sentences	Magnitude	Sentiment score
This drug is absolutely helpful for chest pain.	0.82	+0.555
Last time I'm agonizing because I didn't warm up for swimming activity.	0.85	-0.531
I took mefenamic acid and it didn't work at all.	0.85	-0.531
I can't sleep because of pain in my left chest and back.	0.78	-0.494
I took 40 mg of Aspilet/Aspirin and after few hours, I got relived!	0.49	0.128

positive
negative
neutral

Fig. 8.2 Examples for sentiment analysis on document- and sentence-level. The drug review was processed by the sentiment analyzer provided at: https://text2data.com/Demo. It demonstrates the limitations of document-level sentiment analysis. A human interpreter would classify the review as positive. However, the tool assigned a negative polarity to the entire document. The polarity determined at sentence-level is recognised correctly

is good, but food consumption is limited". The state-of-the art sentence-level analysis tool Text2Data[1] recognises a positive polarity for the term *"good"* and for *"food consumption"* and assigns a positive polarity to the entire sentence. We are missing the different sentiments per topic (drinking behaviour, food consumption). Interestingly, when entering the sentence as two sentences: *"Drinking behaviour is good. But food consumption is limited."* the first sentence is labelled *positive* while the second is correctly classified *negative*.

Holderness et al. tested different sentence-level approaches to determine the polarity of psychiatric EHR texts [87]. When creating their dataset, they ensured that only one aspect (referred to as risk-factor domain in their work) was described in each sentence.

[1] https://text2data.com/Demo.

8.1.3 *Aspect-Level Sentiment Analysis*

Aspect- or topic-level classification can capture a sentiment polarity for each topic or aspect mentioned in a document. An aspect might be a concrete topic, for example a symptom like "headache", or a more broader concept such as "well-being". Consider again the sentence *"Drinking behaviour is good, but food consumption is limited"*. This sentence describes two aspects: "drinking behaviour" and "food consumption". As recognised before, with an aspect-level sentiment approach, polarities expressed towards both aspects can be determined individually. In this sentence, the sentiment expressed regarding "drinking behaviour" is positive while the sentiment towards "food consumption" is negative.

It becomes clear that an analysis on aspect-level helps to detect exactly what people might express towards a particular aspect. This level of analysis would be optimal for sentiment analysis from clinical narratives since it would allow for a detailed assessment of sentiments towards mentioned symptoms, anatomical structures, mental health aspects etc. However, it is the most challenging level of analysis. It requires not only a sentence-level topic detection. Information on the same aspect might be distributed among multiple sentences. Thus, references between sentences have to be recognised by a co-reference resolution method. When two or more aspects are mentioned in a sentence, the corresponding sentiment-bearing terms have to be identified and linked to the correct aspect they refer to. Additional challenges of aspect-level sentiment analysis are described by Nazir et al. [149].

8.2 Tasks Within Medical Sentiment Analysis

When analysing sentiments expressed in medical texts, multiple facets of a medical opinion can be considered. As mentioned before, one initial task is distinguishing subjective from objective sentences, referred to as subjectivity analysis. Subjective pieces of text can express a certain polarity (polarity analysis) and the sentiment can have a particular intensity (intensity classification). More sophisticated medical sentiment analysis methods examine the correlations between the text and various emotional states, including fear, rage, happiness, and sadness (emotion analysis). These different tasks are described in more detail in the following.

8.2.1 *Subjectivity Analysis*

Subjectivity quantifies the amount of opinionated and factual information in a text. An objective sentence basically describes factual information. In contrast, a subjective sentence expresses personal views, feelings, judgements or beliefs, i.e.

opinionated information. Subjectivity detection is an important task within medical sentiment analysis. But, distinguishing objective from subjective sentences with medical content is not always simple. The sentence *"This drug is absolutely helpful for chest pain."* can be considered subjective when it is part of a drug review. It has a positive polarity. When written in a scientific paper *"According to best clinical evidence, this drug is helpful for chest pain"*, we would probably consider it as objective. However, not all subjective sentences necessarily express a positive or negative sentiment (e.g. the subjective sentence *"I need a drug that helps me with my headaches."*).

Further, the definition or characteristics of subjectivity might be different depending on the text source under consideration. When considering medical social media, subjective texts would express opinions of the opinion holders while objective texts will present facts. In this way, subjectivity analysis can help to reduce the volume of data to be processed with follow-up sentiment analysis methods assuming that only subjective texts express sentiments.

In contrast, when considering clinical narratives, many descriptions are observations and could be considered subjective (e.g. the observations of a nurse while caring for a patient or the observations of the radiologist who wrote the finding report based on a radiological image) even though the style of writing is objective. Subjectivity analysis might not be useful in this case.

8.2.2 Polarity Analysis

Another task within sentiment analysis is determining the orientation or polarity of a sentiment, i.e., whether a text expresses a positive, negative or neutral sentiment about the entity in consideration. Sentiment orientation of single words can be identified by sentiment lexicon lookup. From the lexicon entry, the polarity can be retrieved. Another option is to train a classifier for the different polarity classes.

8.2.3 Intensity Classification

Sentiment can have different levels of strength or intensity. Intensity classification is the process of assigning a level of intensity or strength to sentiments. Consider the two sentences: *"I have pain in my knee"* and *"I have a terrible pain in main knee"*. Both sentences specify a negative polarity, but the second sentence expresses it with a higher intensity. From a linguistic point of view, intensity of a sentiment can be expressed using intensifiers such as *very, extremely, terribly*.

There are several ways that intensity can be classified. One common method is to use an ordinal scale, where intensity is ranked on a scale with discrete levels. For example, a scale of 1 to 5 could be used to classify intensity, with 1 being the lowest intensity and 5 being the highest. Another method is to use a continuous scale, where intensity is measured on a continuous range of values. This can be useful for measuring subtle differences in intensity, but can be more challenging to interpret and compare.

Intensity classification is relevant in emotion analysis since also emotions have different strengths (e.g. strong sadness). Additionally, we can consider the problem of distinguishing the certainty level, e.g. the certainty of a diagnosis, as part of intensity classification. Certainty is something specific within medical sentiment analysis. In clinical narratives, certainties are frequently used. They reflect the clinical decision making process, starting from hypotheses and symptoms to even more concrete diagnoses: at the beginning of the diagnostic process, a physician would write *"Suspicion of heart failure disease"*, while after several confirmatory examinations the phrase would be rather *"Diagnosis: Heart failure disease"*. An intensity classifier could assign a lower intensity to the first phrase and a higher intensity to the second when considering the certainty of the diagnosis.

8.2.4 Emotion Recognition

Emotion recognition, as opposed to sentiment analysis, identifies the emotion a person is experiencing or expressing. This emotion is typically categorised as one of several categories, such as joyful, good, angry, sorrowful, fearful, evil, and surprised [186]. Similar to sentiment, emotions can have an intensity (e.g. strong fear or extremely sad). The way someone feels about a subject does not always match their reported sentiment. Therefore, emotion recognition studies different information than sentiment analysis. The following example highlights this.

In the context of COVID-19 pandemic, several researchers applied sentiment analysis and emotion analysis on social media data. With sentiment analysis, they studied the polarities of the statements related to COVID-19; with emotion analysis they learned more about individual‘s feelings in this context. Heras-Pedrosa et al. analysed the crisis communication in the field of public health that has been carried out during the COVID-19 pandemic. They measured the emotions that have been formulated by the population, and related them to the crisis communication strategy that has been carried out by the Spanish Government [43].

Digital health interventions, especially those with conversational user interfaces, may benefit from emotion recognition. A level of empathy from such a system is anticipated that is comparable to the empathy displayed by a healthcare professional during a patient visit. It has been shown that having strong emotional intelligence has a number of beneficial implications on the doctor-patient interaction. Therefore, a digital health intervention needs to be able to identify the user's feelings and emotions in order to respond empathetically, thus, requires emotion analysis methods.

Chapter 9
Document Pre-processing

9.1 Overview

The process of extracting and analysing medical sentiments expressed in a text comprises several steps that are shown in Fig. 9.1. First, data has to be collected from the source under consideration. As described in Part II this data can be retrieved from multiple sources including clinical sources, web sources or even apps and software systems. Once the text is available, it is processed using natural language processing (NLP) techniques. This processing comprises feature extraction including part-of-speech tagging, negation detection and feature selection.

When considering sentiment on aspect-level, aspects or topics mentioned in the text have to be determined and classified. The final sentiment classification is conducted on the extracted and selected features and can be performed using different sentiment analysis approaches (see Chaps. 10 and 11). There are several tools available to realise the single steps. It has to be noted that applying out-of-the-box tools for medical sentiment analysis including the pre-processing steps can result in low quality results. Careful selection of tools including an analysis of their quality when applied to medical text or the development of methods that address the peculiarities of medical text is advised.

9.2 Data Collection and Preparation

Before sentiment of a text can be analysed, the textual data to be analysed has to be collected. Referring to the use cases described before, data sources for medical sentiment analysis can be social media, websites with reviews, clinical notes, transcripts of conversational agents etc. Accordingly, the data collecting methods differ. Web data can be collected using web scraping, i.e. by automatically extracting data from websites. When considering web or social media data, it would be

K. Denecke, *Sentiment Analysis in the Medical Domain*,
https://doi.org/10.1007/978-3-031-30187-2_9

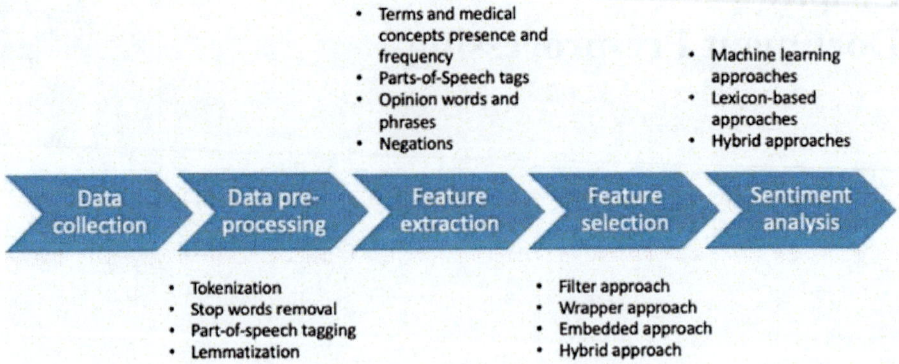

Fig. 9.1 Five sentiment analysis steps together with subtasks

necessary to detect spam in the collected data. Some effort has to be taken to collect the actual text and remove advertisements, etc. Some social media provider offer APIs such as Twitter or Reddit which facilitate collection of tweets and Reddit posts. However, there might be restrictions in the amount of data that can be collected. The maximum number of requests towards the Twitter API that are allowed is based on a time interval, some specified period or window of time.

Clinical narratives cannot be collected without significant effort except the sentiment analysis technology is part of the hospital information system. They are captured in the hospital information system and are legally protected given the sensitive data they contain. For running experiments related to medical sentiment analysis, researchers considered small datasets that have been anonymised or relied upon the datasets presented in Part II. For analysing conversations with intelligent agents in healthcare settings, sentiment analysis methods have to be integrated into the system. Then, the user input can be directly analysed by the sentiment analysis method and an appropriate reaction of the intelligent agent can be generated.

9.3 Text Normalisation

A first step after retrieving textual data is text normalisation. There may be noise, spelling, or grammar errors in the raw text that was acquired using data collecting techniques and technologies. Prior to analysis, text has to be cleaned up and pre-processed by text normalisation. Normalising text means converting it to a more standard form [103]. This pre-processing is supposed to improve the quality of the analysis. One step includes structuring a text into sentences referred to as sentence splitting or sentence segmentation. A second step, referred to as tokenisation, is separating or tokenising words from a text. Stop words are removed from a text since they often do not contribute to the analysis of sentiment. Stop words are terms that are either used a lot in a text or have no discernible significance.

Another step within text normalisation is lemmatisation. This step analyses whether two words have the same root. For example the words *freezes*, *froze* and *frozen* are forms of the verb *freeze*, which is the lemma of these words. Lemmatisation (or morphological analysis) is essential when processing morphological complex languages. A simple form of lemmatisation is stemming. Within stemming, only the suffixes are removed from the end of a word. For example, from the word *diabetic*, the ending "-ic" is removed by a stemmer. In this way, words with the same morphological root can be equally considered. A sentiment lexicon for example cannot contain all morphological variations of a term. Stemming or a morphological analysis of an input text helps in standardising the words and supports successful matching with terms in a sentiment lexicon.

During parts-of-speech (POS) tagging, parts-of-speeches are assigned to each word of an input text. Parts-of-speech include nouns, verbs, pronouns, prepositions, adverbs, conjunctions, particles, and articles. Based on a sequence of tokenised words and a tagset (i.e. a set of possible tags), a part-of-speech tag is assigned to each token. Linguistic ambiguities of words have to solved in this step. There are several tools and programming libraries provided that realise parts-of-speech tagging, for example the Natural Language Toolkit (NLTK[1]). In addition to a collection of text processing libraries for categorisation, tokenisation, stemming, tagging, parsing, and semantic reasoning, as well as wrappers for powerful NLP libraries, NLTK offers simple interfaces to more than 50 corpora and lexical resources, including WordNet.

9.4 Feature Extraction

Feature extraction is a fundamental task in medical sentiment analysis. The considered features can impact on the quality of the sentiment classification. Feature extraction aims at extracting valuable information, e.g. words or concepts that express a sentiment or impact on the sentiment expressed by other words. For this reason, feature extraction is also referred to as text representation: the text is represented by its most characteristic features. In contrast to general domain sentiment analysis, in medical sentiment analysis we have to consider peculiarities of medical texts when extracting features (see Part II).

Some important features or text representations for realising medical sentiment analysis include:

- **Presence of terms and their frequency**: One possibility for text representation is to consider single words and their frequency. Words can be used as features in

[1] https://www.nltk.org.

the form of unigram, bi-gram or n-gram together with their frequency counts in a document. Instead of counting the occurrence of a term or n-gram, its presence could be considered as text representation which would be a binary value (yes, no). Instead of representing a text by all its words, parts-of-speech or specific terms can be considered as outlined in the following items.

- **Parts-of-speech tags**: are labels assigned to words to specify their syntactic function in a sentence. Some sentiment analysis approaches concentrate on terms who are supposed to bear subjectivity, i.e. adjectives. Thus, a text could be represented by counts of adjectives or by counts or frequencies of its parts-of-speech.
- **Opinion words and phrases**: are words and phrases that express sentiments. These words and phrases can be identified using sentiment lexicons. Again, frequency or presence of opinion words and phrases can be used to represent texts.
- **Presence of medical entities and their frequency**: Instead of representing a text by all of its words, a specific focus could be on medical entities. For extracting medical entities, named entity recognition methods have to be applied.

These features do not have to be considered independently, but they can be combined as text or content representation for medical sentiment analysis. Text as basis for sentiment analysis requires often a transformation into a fixed-length feature vector to be able to apply sentiment analysis algorithms. This representation of text is based on the bag of words model or on distributed representations.

9.4.1 Bag of Words

Traditional representations for machine learning exploit bags of words: a vocabulary of all the unique words in the corpus is generated and each word is represented as vector of 0s and 1s where the dimension corresponding to the word is set to 1. For better representation, 0s and 1s can be replaced by better measures such as word frequency, n-grams, parts-of-speech frequencies, TF-IDF-measure etc. as has been outlined before.

9.4.2 Distributed Representation

Distributed representations or embeddings are distributed vector representations that map text to dense fixed length vectors and capture prior knowledge. This means the information about a word or concept is distributed along a vector. Embeddings are induced from large unlabelled corpora (unsupervised learning) and can address the challenge of having a large set of unlabelled data and only a small set of labelled data. They can be classified as prediction-based models (learn embeddings by predicting target words based on context words or vice versa, e.g. Word2Vec [132], ELMo [160], Fasttext, GloVe, BERT [55]) and count-based models (learn embeddings by leveraging global information such as word context co-occurrence in a corpus, e.g. Doc2Vec, paragraph2Vec).

Word2Vec builds vocabulary out of the corpus and learns word representations by training a three-layered neural network. It offers 2 models: Continuous bag of words (CBOW) and Skip-gram. CBOW learns representations by predicting the target word based on its context words. Skip gram learns representations by predicting each of the context words based on the target word. Parameters of Word2Vec include: embedding size, context size, minimum frequency for a word to be included. There are two options to evaluate generated representations: distance (retrieve the most semantically similar words for a given word with cosine similarity) and analogy (find linguistic regularities). The CBOW model consists of three layers: input, hidden and output layer. The layers are connected by two weight matrices W and W'. The input layer takes the one hot vector representation of the context words as input and the output layer applying a softmax function predicts the one hot vector of the target word. Chen et al. applied Word2Vec vs. Doc2Vec [32] for detecting sentiments in clinical discharge summaries.

FastText is an extension of the Word2Vec model. Each word is treated as a bag of character n-grams. Each character n-gram is mapped to a dense vector and the sum of these dense vectors represent the word. In this way, FastText uses subword information and offers better representations for rare words. FastText can be used for efficient learning of word representations and sentence classification.

In **Global Vectors (GloVe)**, a word occurrence matrix is generated in which rows represent the words and columns represent the context. Each value in the matrix represents how frequently a word co-occurs with a context. Factorization of the word co-occurrence matrix results in a low dimensional matrix where rows represent words and columns represent features. Each row in the low dimensional word-feature matrix represents the dense vector representation of a word where the size of feature can be pre-set to the required value. In contrast to Word2Vec, GloVe uses the global contexts in the form of global co-occurrence statistics.

Identifying a well suited feature set or text representation is a crucial task when developing sentiment analysis methods. For this reason, researchers often run experiments comparing different representations and feature sets. Albornoz et al. [42] compared content-based features (word embeddings, concept embeddings, bag of words), domain-specific features (TFxIDF of UMLS semantic types), positional features, sentiment-based features (number of positive/negative words, emotions expressed, part-of-speech, negation).

Niu et al. considered as features: unigram, bigram, change phrases (specific groups of words that indicate changes, e.g. reduce, decline, fall), negation, and the semantic categories of terms as identified using the UMLS Metathesaurus [151].

9.5 Feature Selection

Extracted features represent the text content. However, features can be relevant, irrelevant or redundant. Feature selection aims at removing irrelevant and redundant features from a set of features. This reduces the size of the feature dimension space which can have a positive effect on the speed of the classification algorithm. Removing irrelevant features also improves accuracy of the sentiment classification. Feature selection techniques can be broadly categorised into supervised and unsupervised feature selection methods. Filter and Wrapper methods are examples of supervised feature selection techniques [123]. Wrapper methods depend on machine learning algorithms. They heuristically select features by measuring the accuracy of a machine learning algorithm trained on the selected feature subset [17]. Filter methods select features based on general characteristics of the training data without applying a machine learning algorithm. Instead, features are ranked by statistical measures such as information gain, document frequency or mutual information [17].

9.6 Topic Detection

Sentiments are often expressed towards a topic. When sentiment analysis is conducted on aspect- (or topic-) level, it is crucial to identify the topic and link it to the expressed sentiment. Realising both, topic detection and sentiment analysis, at the same time turns out to be a problem of multi-label classification and regression. Given the complexity of the label schema, most of the stable methods have used a separate topic recognition logic to detect the topics and another one to recognise the sentiment as a second step.

Medical topic detection can be realised by extracting medical entities such as diagnoses, medical procedures or drugs (named entity recognition). Another approach is to extract concepts. This involves identifying and extracting specific concepts as they are represented in medical ontologies. For this purpose, tools such as MetaMap[2] can be used [3]. MetaMap allows to discover UMLS Metathesaurus concepts referred to in text. It uses a knowledge-intensive approach based on symbolic, natural language processing and computational linguistic techniques.

Topics can also be identified by topic modelling methods such as Latent Dirichlet Allocation (LDA) [18]. LDA assumes that documents are a mixture of topics, and some words have a higher probability of occurring in some topics than others. LDA gives a probability vector for each document belonging to a topic. Bahja et al. introduced a medical sentiment analysis approach that used topic modelling with LDA [7]. A more recent approach to topic modelling is BERTopic. It "leverages transformers and c-TF-IDF to create dense clusters allowing for easily interpretable

[2] https://lhncbc.nlm.nih.gov/ii/tools/MetaMap.html.

topics whilst keeping important words in the topic descriptions" [7]. TF-IDF (term frequency-inverse document frequency) is a popular technique for retrieving the most relevant texts given a term or set of terms. c-TF-IDF identifies the most relevant terms given all of the texts belonging to a cluster.

Chapter 10
Lexicon-Based Medical Sentiment Analysis

10.1 Overview on Lexicon-Based Approaches

Sentiment lexicons use scores to relate words to their sentiment orientation. Some lexicons categorise words into positive and negative polarities. Others offer a more precise classification of the sentiment's strength or intensity (e.g. a real value between −1 and 1 in SentiWordNet). Lexicon-based approaches to sentiment analysis are straightforward rule-based techniques that scan texts for opinion words using a lexicon, classify the text or phrase by averaging the polarity of all matched terms, and then assign a sentiment. Advanced methods take into account many classification rules that incorporate dictionary polarity, negation words, booster words, idioms, emoticons, and mixed viewpoints, to name a few. Pre-processing including tokenisation and stemming is an essential step in advance to allow for lexicon matching. Beyond simple averaging sentiment scores of single words to calculate a sentence or document score, more sophisticated rules or algorithms can be used. They consider weighted measures of word incidence or frequency to score all the opinions in the data.

Lexicon-based approaches do not require any training material; a lexicon of sentiments is sufficient. A disadvantage of this approach is its domain-dependency, since words can have multiple meanings depending on the domain and thus, also multiple sentiment orientations. Domain-specific lexicons can address this problem or lexicon-adaptation approaches such as transfer learning. However, meaning is not only domain-dependent, but also context dependent. Even if a sentiment lexicon contains scores for the different meanings of a word, the context of a word has to be taken into account when matching a word with a lexicon to be able to retrieve the proper meaning. A sentiment lexicon reflecting the emotional valence of the words as they are employed in a particular context would be the optimum course of action in such cases. However, creating such dictionaries is challenging, expensive, and time-consuming because it often requires defining each word's emotional connotations.

K. Denecke, *Sentiment Analysis in the Medical Domain*,
https://doi.org/10.1007/978-3-031-30187-2_10

10.2 Approaches to Lexicon Generation

Sentiment lexicons can be generated in a manual process or semi-automatically. Semi-automatic approaches can be separated into dictionary-based approaches and corpus-based approaches. For manual lexicon generation, three steps should be followed:

1. Characterise the medical sentiment,
2. Identify sentiment bearing words,
3. Assign sentiment labels to the words.

These three steps were realised in a manual process by Holderness et al. [87] and Deng et al. [53]. Even though this process is resource intensive, the result is a consistent and reliable sentiment lexicon. Since the sentiment-bearing terms and polarity can be specific to a medical field, it is important to clearly define the considered sentiment before generating a sentiment lexicon. Sentiment bearing words can be identified by corpus annotation where terms and phrases that express the defined sentiment are identified, marked and a polarity or sentiment class is assigned.

Dictionary-based methods for creating sentiment lexicons are predicated on the notion that words with the same meanings bear the same polarity, but words with opposite meanings bear opposite polarities [7]. These methods are based on already existing dictionaries like WordNet or other thesaurus. A list of seed words with known orientation is manually compiled from these dictionaries. By looking up synonyms and antonyms in other lexical resources, this list is widened. The matches are incrementally added to the list. The problem with applying this approach to the medical domain is, that there are only limited lexical resources for medical sentiment analysis that can serve as a seed list. Polarities can also change depending on the medical subdomain.

In contrast to dictionary-based approaches, corpus-based approaches base upon a domain-specific dataset. These approaches try to find co-occurrence patterns in the corpus. They start from a list of seed sentiment words with known polarity and exploit co-occurrence patterns to find new sentiment words in a corpus of texts. To assign polarity, the principle of sentiment consistency is used (e.g. two adjectives connected by the conjunction "and" have most probably the same polarity).

Approaches where medical sentiment lexicons have been developed are still rare. Liu and Lee applied word embeddings to SentiWordNet to generate an enhanced sentiment lexicon for the medical domain [117]. A corpus of clinical narratives is used for training a medical domain specific Word2Vec model. Sentiment phrases that appear frequently in clinical narratives, but are not included in SentiWordNet are discovered by similarity measurements. They are stored in a domain specific sentiment lexicon. Polarities are gathered using rules from a corpus of drug reviews.

The medical sentiment lexicon SentiHealth [5] was developed using bootstrapping, a dataset of health reviews, and corpus-based sentiment detection and scoring. Vocabulary of the lexicon was updated iteratively starting from an initial seed cache. Irrelevant words were filtered out, and a sentiment class and score were assigned to each word (see Chap. 7).

Chapter 11
Machine Learning-Based Sentiment Analysis Approaches

11.1 Unsupervised Learning Approaches

We already recognised that labelled training data is very rare in the field of medical sentiment analysis. Reason is that the generation process requires people labelling data which is labour-intensive and time-consuming. Additionally, due to data privacy issues it is very difficult to published datasets with clinical narratives even though they have been anonymised. Unsupervised learning approaches to medical sentiment analysis do not depend on labelled datasets. They make use of the statistical properties captured in texts and corpora. These properties include word co-occurrence, frequencies of words or of sentiment-bearing terms (see feature extraction in Sect. 9.4). Unsupervised approaches to medical sentiment analysis use clustering methods, which can group data into clusters without explicitly specifying the sentiment or polarity of the data elements in a cluster. The data elements in one cluster are similar from a particular point of view, i.e. they share common features. Clustering methods can be grouped into partition methods and hierarchical methods.

11.1.1 Partition Methods

Partition methods for clustering group data into a set of non-overlapping clusters where each data element is assigned only to one cluster. Based on a similarity criterion, such as the Euclidean distance between elements, the partitioning is performed. Data within one cluster has a short distance to elements of the same cluster while having a large distance to data elements of another cluster.

K-means clustering is a well-known partitioning technique used, among other things, for medical sentiment analysis. This approach begins with a predetermined number of initial cluster centroids and iteratively allocates each dataset's data elements to a cluster centroid based on the similarity between the data element and

K. Denecke, *Sentiment Analysis in the Medical Domain*,
https://doi.org/10.1007/978-3-031-30187-2_11

the cluster centroids. When the outcome remains the same after a predetermined number of iterations, the procedure ends.

Hussein et al. used k-means clustering for exploring COVID-19 pandemic sentiment expressed in tweets [93]. The textual data was pre-processed, i.e. punctuation, stopwords and special characters were removed and terms were extracted using the Term Frequency-Inverse Document Frequency (TF-IDF) technique. To reduce irrelevant features, the Singular Value Decomposition (SVD) technique was used. The tweets were divided into 9 groups by k-means clustering. The polarity of the tweets belonging to the same cluster was calculated to estimate the sentiment of each cluster. Each tweet in the sample was given a polarity score using the tool TextBlob (see Sect. 12.2). The sentiment of a cluster was defined as the sentiment average across all tweets in that cluster. Worth mentioning, that it is unclear if tweets were grouped together in one cluster due to a shared topic or due to a common sentiment because no sentiment-specific characteristics were utilised. The k-means clustering technique itself does not perform the actual sentiment analysis.

11.1.2 Hierarchical Clustering Methods

Besides partition methods for clustering, other types of methods for clustering exist. Hierarchical methods create a cluster having a tree-type structure (i.e. groups that have sub-groups). Strategies to hierarchical clustering can be divided into two main strategies: agglomerative (bottom-up approach) and divisive (top-down approach) clustering approaches.

The agglomerative clustering method initially treats each data item as its own cluster. At each step of the algorithm, the two clusters that are most similar are combined into a new bigger cluster. This procedure is iterated until all points are member of just one single big cluster. The result is a tree-based representation of the data objects, named dendrogram. Its leaves are the single-element clusters; the nodes the aggregated cluster. For measuring the similarity of two clusters, the Euclidean distance or another distance measure can be used.

The divisive clustering first considers the entire data as one cluster and then segments this cluster into smaller sub-clusters through a recursive process. At each step of iteration, the most heterogeneous cluster is divided into two.

11.2 Supervised Approaches

Supervised approaches to medical sentiment analysis exploit models trained from labelled corpora. Four types of supervised classification approaches are distinguished: linear, probabilistic, rule-based methods, and decision tree. Supervised classification algorithms include Support Vector Machines (SVM), Naive Bayes, Logistic regression [75], based-BiLSTM [77], Decision tree, k-Nearest Neighbours, Logistic regression, Stochastic gradient descent [89]. The use of supervised techniques for medical sentiment analysis is detailed in the sections that follow, along with examples. The relevant machine learning literature can be accessed for thorough descriptions of the underlying mathematics and techniques.

11.2.1 Linear Approaches

A statistical method known as linear classification bases its classification decision on a linear combination of the feature vector of a text. For a two-class classification problem, the operation of a linear classifier can be compared to splitting a high-dimensional input space with a hyperplane. Hyperplanes are decision boundaries that help classify the data points, i.e. all points on one side of the hyperplane are classified as "yes", while the others are classified as "no". A linear classifier is used in situations where the speed of classification matters, since it is often the fastest classifier while achieving state-of-the-art performances when appropriate features are used.

Support vector machines (SVM) belong to the linear approaches of machine learning that can handle discrete and continuous variables. An SVM-based classifier aims at finding a hyperplane in an N-dimensional space that distinctly classifies the data points—with N as the number of features. More specifically, it is seeking the hyperplane that maximises the margin of separation between the objects belonging to two different classes.

This algorithm has frequently been used for medical sentiment analysis. Jiménez-Zafra et al. studied sentiments in medical forums in Spanish [97]. They compared various feature sets (TFxIDF, TF, Word2Vec, Binary term occurrences[1]) and applied an SVM classifier. As baseline they used a lexicon-based approach. Depending on the corpus and features used, they achieved accuracy values between 64% and 87%, outperforming the lexicon-based approach.

Niu et al. [151] assessed the polarity of clinical outcomes and divided them into four categories *no outcomes, positive outcomes, negative outcomes*, and *neutral outcomes*. When using SVM, they compared the performance of several feature set combinations, including unigrams, bigrams, change phrases, negations, and UMLS semantic categories. They showed that the linguistic and domain knowledge features work well together to produce accurate classification results of outcome polarity (achieving a precision of 86%).

Mishra et al. [133] used drug reviews written by patients derived from various health communities to judge the performance of a drug. The dataset was annotated using crowdsourcing. The review-level, sentence-level, and aspect-level of senti-

[1] Within the weighting scheme Binary term occurrences each term receives a value of 1 if it is present in the document or a value of 0 otherwise.

ment analysis were all taken into consideration and sentiment was classified using an SVM classifier.

11.2.2 Probabilistic Approaches

A probabilistic classifier such as Naïve Bayes or Maximum entropy predicts a probability distribution over a set of classes. Naïve Bayes is a machine learning classifier that is often used for text classification tasks. The machine learning model is based on the Bayes Theorem and word frequencies are used as features. The position of a word and its context are ignored with this approach.

The Naïve Bayes algorithm was used to categorise emotions in suicide notes [180] with an F-measure of 53%. Lexical resources (SentiWordNet, WordNet-Affect, and the Macquarie Semantic Orientation Lexicon) and pattern matching were used to extract the features.

Maximum entropy is a principle used to determine the probability distribution that is most consistent with the available information. It estimates the probability distribution of the class label of a document to maximise the likelihood (entropy). Overall, the maximum entropy principle is a useful tool for making probabilistic predictions in situations where there is incomplete information or uncertainty. A case study analysing Twitter data regarding health conditions and expressed sentiments used a maximum entropy classifier [90]. The classifier was trained on TF-IDF weighted word frequency features.

11.2.3 Rule-Based Classifier

Rule-based classification refers to a sentiment classification approach that uses a set of "if-then" rules for predicting a class. Rules are represented in disjunctive normal form where the *if* clause is referred to as rule antecedent and the *then* clause is called rule consequent of the rule when the antecedent is satisfied [105]. Rule-based classifiers can classify new instances rapidly with a performance comparable to Decision tree classifiers [17].

Khan et al. applied a rule-based classifier to classify user reviews in social media. They identified subjective texts using a lexicon that included emoticons and opinionated words. The actual sentiment classification took into account a rule that makes use of SentiWordNet's polarity values.

11.2.4 Decision Tree Classifier

Within decision tree classifiers the training data space is decomposed hierarchically [17]. The decision tree consists of internal nodes (representing attributes), branches (decision rules), and leaf nodes reflecting the outcomes. From the sentiment classification perspective, the decision rules lead the leaf nodes to whether the sentiment polarity is positive, negative, or neutral [134]. Decision tree classifiers work well on large datasets and are less advisable for small datasets [17].

Anwar et al. compared a decision tree approach to a Naïve Bayes approach to perform sentiment analysis on smoking perceptions made available in social media [134]. As features they used n-grams. The decision tree had significantly higher accuracy than Naïve Bayes when the model was applied to a specific Twitter data set (one-word tweet search).

11.3 Semi-supervised Approaches

Semi-supervised approaches to machine learning are used when there is only limited labelled data available. In these methods, the feature learning process is supervised using a small set of originally labelled training data. By doing so, the approaches shorten the time needed for manually labelling the data while also giving a classifier significant generalisation skills.

Semi-supervised sentiment analysis frequently uses self-training methodologies. Self-training is divided into two stages: The labelled data is used to train the classifier initially. Second, unlabelled data is applied to the trained classifier. An improved classifier is learned by appending the samples with the highest degree of confidence to the labelled training examples. This second phase is iterated upon. The final classifier is applied to the test data.

Reinforcement learning is another semi-supervised approach used within sentiment analysis. It learns from historical experiences to correct errors committed during the training process. More specifically, the algorithm is rewarded based on the performance of the previous action it has made. Thus, this learning algorithm employs a trial-and-error process to decide on actions that assist in maximising rewards.

For the purpose of analysing sentiment in Chinese microblogs, Liu et al. developed a semi-supervised sentiment classification system [119]. They were trying to address the issue of the imbalanced sentiment distribution of microblogs, which results in the minority class receiving poor performance from binary classifiers. Their strategy resembles a self-training method. To compute confidence scores, a set of labelled samples is set aside. Through this procedure, samples that fall below a predetermined confidence score threshold are added to the training set for subsequent training. By doing this, the classifier can improve its performance on samples from the minority class.

Holderness et al. compared three approaches for determining the clinical sentiment connected to single risk factor domains in their paper [86]. As baseline model, they considered a majority vote approach using the Pattern sentiment lexicon employed by McCoy [127] and Waudby-Smith [198]. This baseline model was tested against models built using the multilayer perceptron (MLP) architecture in two different supervision levels: fully supervised and semi-supervised.

11.4 Deep Learning Approaches

Applying deep learning-based approaches on artificial neural networks (ANN) to sentiment analysis became very popular in recent years. Inspired by the construction of the human brain, deep learning refers to neural networks with multiple layers of perceptrons. Deep learning includes various neural network models such as Convolutional Neural Networks (CNN), Recurrent Neural Networks (RNN), or Deep Belief Networks (DBN). These models learn the features from a dataset by themselves. However, the learned models are comprehensive, understandable only to a limited extent by humans and computationally expensive.

11.4.1 Deep Neural Networks (DNN)

DNN are ANN with several hidden layers embedded between the input and output layers [171]. The input layer includes the input data. Hidden layers include the processing nodes. The lower-order layers that are close to the input layer learn trivial features, while higher-order layers learn more significant features obtained from lower layer features. The DNN architecture and its derivations—CNN and RNN—have been used in multiple NLP tasks.

11.4.2 Convolutional Neural Networks (CNN)

The hidden layers of a CNN have three main types, which are: Convolutional layer, pooling layer, fully-connected layer. The convolutional layer is the first layer of a CNN and filters the inputs to extract features (e.g. the word embeddings in sentiment analysis). Pooling layers reduce the resolution of features [17]. Convolutional layers can be followed by additional convolutional layers or pooling layers. The fully-connected layer is the final layer used to perform the classification task.

A CNN was tested by Colón-Ruiz et al. for sentiment analysis on drug reviews [37]. Their CNN architecture has "a convolution layer, where different filters operate sliding along the matrix of word embeddings of each drug review, producing as output a mapping of features of the reviews" [37]. The architecture is composed of

64 filters with a window size of 2, 3 and 5-word vectors. Linear rectification unit (ReLU) is used as activation function. In terms of training time, CNN outperformed LSTM or hybrid models.

Yadav et al. used CNN for extracting sentiments from users' posts in medical blogs [204]. Their architecture consisted of an input layer, a word embedding layer that encodes each word into a real-valued vector, a convolutional layer, a pooling layer and an output layer. It achieved F1-Scores between 63-81%.

11.4.3 Long Short-Term Memory (LSTM)

LSTM is a special type of recurrent neural network (RNN) that has feedback connections and extends the "short" memory of RNN. A bidirectional LSTM was the basis of the method utilised by Colón-Ruiz et al. [37]. Long-term dependencies and contextual information can both be captured by this kind of RNN. The bidirectional LSTM of Colón-Ruiz et al. has a hidden state dimension of 250 for the forward and backward layers and a hyperbolic tangent (tanh) as activation function.

Mohan et al. considered the problem of detecting depressions using a combination of results from analysing facial expressions and sentiment of user texts. They used an architecture consisting of an embedding layer, an LSTM layer and a dense layer with softmax as activation function as output layer [140] for analysing the sentiment of user texts.

11.5 Hybrid Approaches

Combining two or more approaches to sentiment analysis is referred to as hybrid approach. Colón-Ruiz et al. suggested such hybrid approach by combining CNN with bidirectional LSTM [37]: The CNN architecture (see section before) is used to extract a sequence of representations of higher-level texts which are conformed by the concatenation of the pooling layers. The result is used to feed a bidirectional LSTM to capture contextual information from the local features.

Using a dataset of psychosis patient discharge summaries and the Pattern lexical opinion mining lexicon, McCoy et al. employed a majority vote classifier to categorise the related sentiment of documents [127]. A voting classifier is a type of machine learning estimator that develops a number of base models or estimators and makes predictions based on averaging their results.

Another example for a hybrid approach to affective computing and sentiment analysis is Sentic computing. It exploits both knowledge-based methods and statistical methods to perform emotion recognition and detect sentiments in natural language text [26].

11.6 Concluding Remarks

The landscape of machine learning algorithms is huge; even more methods exist than have been introduced in this chapter. I was focusing on methods that have been reported in research papers on medical sentiment analysis. However, we can recognise that at the time of publishing this book, in particular for sentiment analysis from clinical narratives, only few machine learning methods have been tested. Deep learning algorithms are rising techniques in sentiment analysis in other domains [112]. Attention mechanism (self attention [113]), transformer-based models and gated multiplication (Gated CNN [203]) are widely used to realise sentiment analysis in the general domain, i.e. outside the medical context. However, those newly emerged methods have not yet been tested with clinical narratives.

One reason might be that large repositories of data are missing in the medical sentiment analysis domain that are needed for training classifiers or learning statistical models. Another reason might be that medical sentiment analysis is still at its beginnings and not all approaches have been studied in sufficient detail yet. A majority of existing papers on medical sentiment analysis is using ready-to-use tools for sentiment analysis, resisting on a domain-specific adaptation. This can be sufficient, however, most papers resisted on studying the quality of the sentiment analysis tools they applied to their data. I conclude, that there are still many open research questions that can be tackled in the context of medical sentiment analysis, in particular for clinical narratives. An outline is given in Chap. 18.

Chapter 12
Sentiment Analysis Tools

12.1 Sentiment 140 Sentiment Analysis Tool

Sentiment140 is a machine learning-based algorithm that allows to discover the sentiment of a topic on Twitter [72]. The researcher who developed that tool compared different bag of words feature sets (unigrams, bigrams, unigrams and bigrams, and unigrams with part-of-speech tags) and tested three different classifiers (Naïve Bayes, Maximum Entropy, Support Vector Machine). Depending on feature set and classification algorithm, the classifier achieved an accuracy between 79% and 82.7%.

The training data was automatically created. The approach based upon the assumption that any tweet with positive emoticons, like *":)"*, is positive, and tweets with negative emoticons, like *":("*, are negative. The Twitter Search API was used to collect these tweets by using keyword search [72]. Developers of the Sentiment140 sentiment analysis tool provide an API which allows to integrate this sentiment analysis classifier into own applications and use it for data analysis.

12.2 TextBlob

TextBlob[1] is an open source Python library for processing textual data. It provides a simple API for realising NLP tasks including part-of-speech tagging, noun phrase extraction, sentiment analysis, and classification. TextBlob contains two sentiment analysis implementations: One is based on the Pattern library (see below); the other one is based on the natural language toolkit (NLTK). NLTK uses statistical approaches and regular expressions to determine the polarity and subjectivity of

[1] https://textblob.readthedocs.io/en/dev/.

K. Denecke, *Sentiment Analysis in the Medical Domain*,
https://doi.org/10.1007/978-3-031-30187-2_12

a given text. The values are based on the adjectives appearing in a text. They are optimised based on the frequency of the adjectives and successive words. The NLTK sentiment classifier is trained on a movie reviews corpus which has to be kept in mind when using this classifier for medical sentiment analysis. TextBlob was used by Waudby et al. to extract sentiment and attitudes of nurses [198] and by Subirats et al. [185]. Zou et al. used TextBlob to support mortality risk prediction for patients with Sepsis [210].

12.3 Pattern for Python

The Pattern library[2] is a library capable of realising NLP tasks such as tokenization, stemming, parts-of-speech tagging, sentiment analysis, data mining and machine learning [44]. Pattern‘s sentiment method assigns a polarity (i.e. a sentiment score between 1 and -1) to the input text as well as a subjectivity value between 0 and 1. Pattern contains a lexicon comprising adjectives and adverbs in English, each of which is mapped to "polarity", "subjectivity" and "intensity" scores. Given a string of text, Pattern uses a POS tagger to identify adjectives and adverbs whose polarity, subjectivity, and intensity scores are retrievable from the lexicon. Pattern was compared to other tools by Weismann et al. by applying it to clinical notes associated with patients with an intensive care unit stay [199].

12.4 Valence Aware Dictionary and Sentiment Reasoner (VADER)

VADER is a lexicon and rule-based sentiment analysis tool that is specifically designed to analyse sentiments expressed in social media [94]. It is fully open-sourced under the MIT License. VADER incorporates a sentiment lexicon that is especially attuned to microblog-like contexts. It was empirically validated by multiple independent human judges. The VADER sentiment lexicon is sensitive to both, the polarity and the intensity of sentiments expressed in social media contexts, and is also generally applicable to sentiment analysis in other domains. It calculates a score by summing the valence scores of each word in the lexicon, adjusted according to defined rules, and then normalised to be between -1 (most extreme negative) and +1 (most extreme positive).

VADER was used to calculate daily and average sentiment scores for topics identified in tweets from Ontario, Canada, during the second wave of the COVID-19 pandemic [190]. Raghupathi et al. applied VADER to study the public perception about vaccination expressed in tweets [162].

[2] https://github.com/clips/pattern.

12.5 TensiStrength

TensiStrength is a system to detect strength of stress and relaxation expressed in text. It relies upon a lexicon-based approach and provides a list of terms related to stress and relaxation. Its emotion terms were obtained from SentiStrength[3] [131]. Stress terms and indicators of stressors and stressful situations were collected from several social media sources. Each term has a numerical strength rating from 1 (no relaxation) to 5 (highly relaxed) for relaxation and from -1 (no stress) to -5 (very high stress) for stress. The sentiment lookup table integrated in the tool is a list of stress or relaxation terms together with their value of strength. It can be easily adapted. TensiStrength was originally developed for English and optimised for general short social web texts, such as tweets. It was used to understand and measure psychological stress using social media [80].

12.6 LIWC

Linguistic Inquiry and Word Counts (LIWC) is a tool for automated text analysis. It calculates the degree to which various categories of words are used in text. It includes several dictionaries (see Sect. 7.1) that form the basis of the analysis. LIWC reads a given text and compares each word in the text to the list of dictionary words and calculates the percentage of total words in the text that match each of the dictionary categories. An example is shown in Table 12.1. A Reddit post was analysed by the LIWC demo app. LIWC shows the percentage of words of the post belonging to the different LIWC dimensions. A comparison value is also shown for the specific text type under consideration (in the example social media). It can be seen that there are much more terms referring to cognitive processes in the analysed text than usual in average social media.

12.7 Other Tools

Beyond the tools described before, more are available. The commercial tool RapidMiner[4] was used by Pandesenda et al. to study service quality of online healthcare platforms [156]. Semantria from Lexalytics[5] is a commercial sentiment engine. It returns both the score and a three-point scale of negative, neutral and positive. It was used by Grissette et al. to study sentiments in drug reviews [78].

[3] http://sentistrength.wlv.ac.uk.

[4] https://rapidminer.com.

[5] https://semantria-docs.lexalytics.com/docs.

Table 12.1 LIWC analysis result generated using the LIWC app demo available at https://www.liwc.app/demo-results. Input text is the Reddit post in Fig. 3.2. LIWC also shows values for comparison for this particular type of language (social media language)

Traditional LIWC dimension	Your text	Average for social media language
I-words (I, me, my)	4.97	5.44
Positive Tone	4.35	5.93
Negative Tone	2.48	2.34
Social words	5.59	6.74
Cognitive Processes	19.25	8.86
Allure	8.07	8.62
Moralization	0.00	0.27
Summary variables		
Analytic	13.59	47.06
Authentic	44.74	62.38

SEANCE[6] is a sentiment analysis tool that relies on a number of preexisting sentiment, social-positioning, and cognition dictionaries [40].

sentimentr is designed to quickly calculate text polarity in the English language at sentence-level and to optionally aggregate it by rows or grouping variables [165]. It uses a dictionary lookup approach that tries to incorporate weighting for valence shifters (negation and amplifiers/deamplifiers). Weissmann et al. compared sentimentr with results from other sentiment analysis tools when applying to text of encounter notes of patients with critical illness [199]. Among the other tools are CoreNLP's sentiment annotator, which uses a deep neural network approach to build up sentiment representation of a sentence on top of its grammatical structure [178]. KNIME Analytics Platform[7] is an open source software for data science. It is based on a graphical user interface for visual programming. It has been designed to be open to different data formats, data types, data sources, data platforms. It also includes a number of extensions for the analysis of unstructured data, like texts or graphs. For text processing, the KNIME Text Processing extension offers a wide variety of input/output options and methods for data cleaning, processing, stemming, or keyword extraction.

[6] https://www.linguisticanalysistools.org/seance.html.

[7] https://www.knime.com.

Chapter 13
Case Studies

13.1 Learning About Suicidal Ideation

13.1.1 The Problem

Suicide is one of the leading causes of death in the world. To prevent an individual of committing suicide his or her pronunciations of suicide or associated feelings have to be recognised. Suicide can be prevented if the signs and clues are recognised right at their beginning. To perform a better risk assessment, suicide prevention researchers analyse patient histories, statements in social media, and suicide notes. However, given the volume of such textual data, a manual analysis is time consuming.

13.1.2 Solution Overview

Feelings or pronunciations of suicide expressed by individuals can be assessed from different sources. With the increased popularity of social media, such as Facebook, Twitter, Reddit, and Tumblr, Internet users are now sharing their suicidal feelings and thoughts on these platforms. Their postings tell a lot about the emotion of an individual, whether he or she feels bored, annoyed, sad, neutral or depressed. From these data sources, text messages can be identified that express suicidal ideations [2] using sentiment analysis techniques. The analysis provides patterns, relevant text snippets or polarity scores for manual assessment or further automatic processing.

K. Denecke, *Sentiment Analysis in the Medical Domain*,
https://doi.org/10.1007/978-3-031-30187-2_13

13.1.3 Methods and Procedures

The overall design of a system that analyses suicidal ideations is shown in Fig. 13.1. The goal of the automatic processing is to provide text snippets together with identified emotions and patterns for manual assessment. Additionally, the recognised patterns can be used as features for predicting a suicide risk score. Methods for text analysis and sentiment analysis are used along with document-gathering methods to identify and classify sentiments in social media postings. These methods can be grouped into the following components:

- A Web crawler fetches postings from dedicated social media channels such as suicide forums. The collected documents are cleaned and stored for further analysis.
- Sentiment analysis techniques process the documents. Features are extracted such as opinionated words, parts-of-speech etc. These features are exploited by clustering algorithms to identify patterns in the data or by machine learning algorithms to distinguish texts containing suicide ideations from those without and to classify sentiments and emotions. Pattern could reveal specific vocabulary that can be associated with an increased suicide risk. This feature information can be further used by a prediction algorithm to calculate a suicide risk score.
- The results of the sentiment analysis are presented for human assessment. Words or phrases expressing suicide ideation are highlighted; an emotion score and a suicide risk score are shown.

An example implementation for detecting suicidal ideation in online forums was presented by Alada et al. [2]. They crawled Reddit posts published between 2008 and 2016 on SuicideWatch, Depression, Anxiety, and ShowerThoughts subreddits. A small subset of these postings (785) were randomly selected and were manually annotated as suicidal or non-suicidal. Features were extracted using term frequency-inverse document frequency (TFxIDF); the LIWC 2015 tool (Linguistic Inquiry and Word Count Matrix, LIWC) was used for producing word count matrices and sentiment analysis was realised using Python's TextBlob library. The LIWC 2015 tool produces matrices with word counts. Logistic regression, random forest, and SVM classification algorithms were applied on the feature set. The logistic regression and SVM classifiers identified suicidality of posts with an F1 score of 92% closely followed by random forest with an F1 score of 89%. The baseline was computed using a ZeroR algorithm achieving 66% F1 score [2]. A ZeroR classifier simply predicts the majority category: After constructing a frequency table for the target variable, the most frequent value is selected.

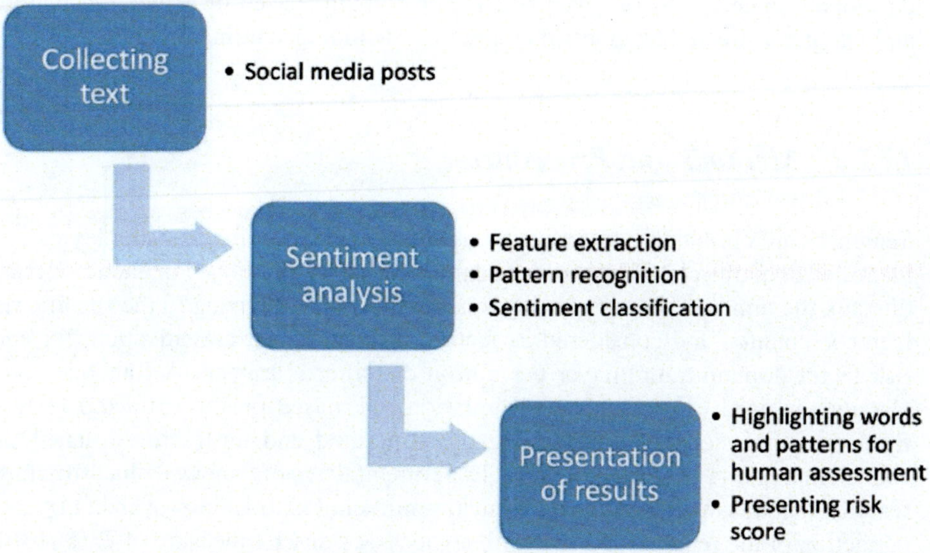

Fig. 13.1 Overview of suicide risk prediction

13.2 Predicting the Psychiatric Readmission Risk

13.2.1 The Problem

Hospital readmissions are a key driver of healthcare costs and avoiding them is crucial to reduce costs and disruptions for patients and their families [130]. Predicting which patients are more likely to be readmitted within 30 days after discharge is important for selecting the treatment interventions and for implementing preventive measures.

The EHR provides information that allows to predict the readmission risk. Approaches that explore structured information from the EHR such as sociodemographic data, comorbidity codes and physiological variables still require qualitative improvements.

13.2.2 Solution Overview

The unstructured data of the EHR (e.g. admission notes, progress notes, discharge summaries) comprises additional information that might be helpful in increasing the quality of the readmission risk prediction. Alvarez-Mellado et al. distinguished seven risk factor domains [130]: Appearance, thought process, thought content, interpersonal, substance use, occupation and mood. The risk prediction model is developed related to these seven risk factor domains based on structured features and features extracted from unstructured data including sentiment polarity.

13.2.3 Methods and Procedures

Sentences are classified into one of the seven risk factor domains using lexicons of identified domain-related keywords and multi-word expressions. For each risk factor domain, the number of sentences in the admission note referring to the specific risk factor is counted and considered as feature. For sentiment classification, for each risk factor domain a multilayer perceptron classifier is trained. A Random Forest classifier is used to predict the readmission risk based on the extracted features from the admission note comprising the structured and unstructured data [130] and including the sentiment scores. Experimental results showed that structured features together with features on clinical sentiment led to an improvement of early prediction of the readmission risk with an accuracy and F1 measure of 72% [130].

13.3 Generating a Corpus for Clinical Sentiment Analysis

13.3.1 The Problem

We want to develop a sentiment analysis method for a specific use case which is studying the patient health status with its facets related to movements, vital signs, anatomy or neurological reactions. For this problem, no labelled training data set is available to train a sentiment classifier [53]. Therefore, a task-specific corpus for sentiment analysis has to be developed.

13.3.2 Solution Overview

A use case specific definition of medical sentiment is developed and expressed in an annotation schema. The annotation schema is used by human annotators to label the sentences of a corpus of clinical notes resulting in an annotated clinical sentiment dataset.

13.3.3 Methods and Procedures

A comprehensive definition for medical sentiment was created. The sentiment objects under consideration relate to fine-grained sentiment aspects of the patient status and their healthcare context. More specifically, clinical sentiment is considered as an event that reflects the patient's body status (referred to as patient status event), coupled with context objects which refer to clinical interventions, pharmaceutical interventions, and social connections (see Fig. 13.2). Besides clinical intervention (e.g. physical therapy, balloon placement), the pharmaceutical therapy is an important measure to support the entire treatment process in clinical care. It can concern for example anaesthesia, pharmaceutical treatment or end of life care. The third type of context objects relate to a patient status indicating a patient‘s social connectedness expressed by relationships, spiritual or religious support and relatives' visiting, which are considered as indicators of the social connectedness. These context objects influence the patient status [53] and provide important context information for judging the patient status.

The patient‘s body status or patient status event refers to descriptions and judgements related to the parts of body, movement capabilities, input and output of patients as well as the vital signs, emotions and feelings (see Fig. 13.2). Typically, the author of a clinical text directly expresses polarity to show the attitude towards the patient status and its elements. Consider the following example for a patient status event: *Multiple blisters on the trunk/chest , oozing from the swollen scrotum.* In this phrase, the author refers to anatomical signs: the patient status event is expressed by the anatomical terms *blisters, trunk, chest, scrotum.* Polarity is

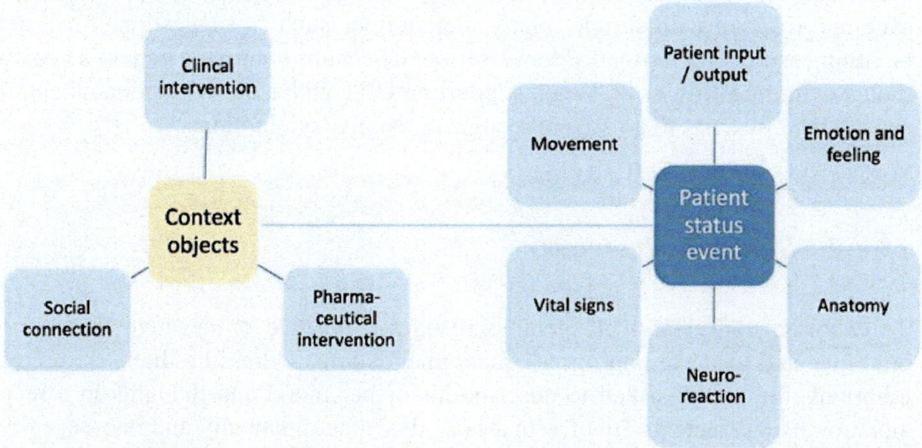

Fig. 13.2 Annotation schema for context objects and patient status event [53]. Clinical sentiment is considered an event that reflects the patient‘s body status coupled with context objects. Context objects can have a positive or negative impact on the patient status event. A patient status event can be positive, negative or neutral

expressed by *multiple, oozing, swollen* resulting in a negative polarity for this (anatomical) patient status event.

Polarity is associated with the patient status. Three sentiment values (positive, negative, neutral) are annotated with respect to the patient status event. The context objects additionally influence the patient status and the entire polarity outcome. Their polarity is limited to two categories: positive and negative, since a neutral polarity would mean that there is no impact of the context object to the outcome. The polarity of the patient status events together with the polarity of the impacting context objects form an aggregated polarity.

Consider another example sentence with a context object concerning the social connections of a patients: *Family called in the middle of night and in to see pt. Priest called in and last rights given.* There is no specific patient status event, but the phrases are just referring to the patient. The family that called in the middle of the night as well as the priest to whom the last rights were given, indicate a negative context. The polarity of these phrases aggregate to negative.

This medical sentiment definition was used to annotate 300 nurse letters from an intensive care unit derived from the MIMIC-II database provided by Deng et al. [53].

13.4 Conversational Agent with Emotion Recognition

13.4.1 The Problem

Individuals having problems in regulating their emotions are treated with cognitive behaviour therapy (CBT). Within CBT it is vital to understand the emotional state and respond with simple micro-interventions such as suggestions for a deep breathing exercise or a friendly conversation. CBT aims to turn the patient's negative thoughts into positive ones. When supporting CBT with a conversational agent, the system therefore has to be able to recognise feelings or emotions.

13.4.2 Solution Overview

To enable a conversational agent to recognise positive or negative thoughts or emotions and to make appropriate recommendations addressing the user's current emotions, the user is asked to describe his or her mood and thoughts in a recent situation using freetext. This freetext is analysed automatically and one out of five core emotions (fear, anger, grief, sadness, joy) is assigned automatically. The user is asked for verifying the detected emotion before corresponding micro-interventions are suggested.

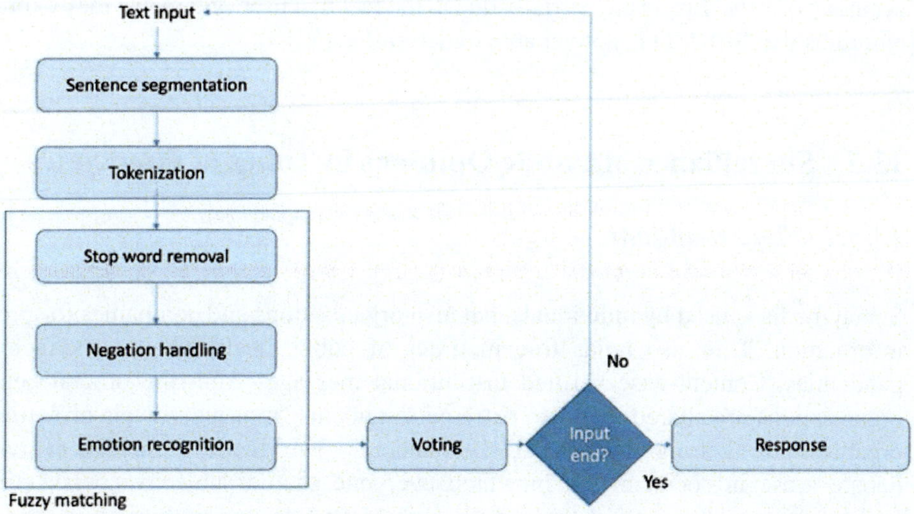

Fig. 13.3 Emotion analysis process in SERMO

13.4.3 Methods and Procedures

A system that realises this solution is SERMO [52]. Its implemented emotion analysis algorithm consists of six steps and uses a lexicon-based approach (see Fig. 13.3). First, the user input is split into sentences which are tokenised in a second step. Third, stop words are removed, i.e. all words that are irrelevant for emotion classification. This includes prepositions, pronouns etc. Fourth, negations are detected to invert the meaning of negated emotion words. Fifth, the emotion terms are determined and finally, the input is classified into one out of the five emotion categories. The underlying emotion lexicon is the Emotional Dictionary of SentiWS. The SentiWS is a publicly available German vocabulary for emotion analysis [163]. It covers the five emotions listed above. In order to deal with typos and writing errors, a fuzzy matching method is used for identifying emotion terms within the lexicon [31]. In this way, words can be recognised even if they are linguistic variations of a word in the dictionary.

For the user input, all matches of terms with the emotion lexicon are determined. Per emotion class, the number of terms that have been identified are calculated. Finally, the user input is classified as emotion class where the largest number of terms were extracted from the input. In some cases, however, it may happen that no emotion terms are identified or there is no majority of emotion terms of one specific category. In these cases, the application responds that it could not identify the user's emotion and asks the user to select one of the five emotions he or she can identify with. Depending on the determined or selected emotion, the dialogue proceeds as foreseen in the emotion-specific dialogues. The emotion classification achieves an accuracy of 81%. Errors are partially due to the fact that user statements may express emotions that SERMO is not yet able to determine [52].

13.5 Surveillance of Public Opinions in Times of Pandemics

13.5.1 The Problem

Social media is used by individuals, but also organisations and companies to spread information. This also holds true in times of public health challenges such as pandemics. Content-wise verified institutional messages from the official health organisations are shared, but also extreme statements from individuals or extreme organisations. During the COVID-19 pandemic worldwide a rapidly evolving debate arose in social media in which everyone shared subjective perspectives (either positive or negative), mixed-up with legitimate and authoritative sources of information [39]. This led to community anxiety and emotional contagion, strengthened by the fact that people tend to hear and share opinions that are similar to their own. In this context, a timely evaluation of the sentiment and emotional contagion on social media becomes useful to be able to develop potential preventive strategies and inform the population correctly.

13.5.2 Solution Overview

Data from Twitter as a huge source of social media content is collected for a specific period of time (if done retrospectively; otherwise continuously). Relevant tweets are gathered by employing specific hashtags such as *#coronavirus* or related keywords. A social media analysis is conducted considering sentiment and longitudinal trends by applying emotion and sentiment analysis tools [39].

13.5.3 Methods and Procedures

In the study under consideration here, features related to emotion and sentiment expressed in tweets were identified by performing sentiment analysis, by using both, (1) the dictionary VADER [94] (Valence Aware Dictionary for Sentiment Reasoning) and the CT-BERT: Covid Twitter BERT (Bidirectional Encoder Representations from Transformers) model [145]; and (2) emotion analysis using the NRC Word-Emotion Association Lexicon (EmoLex, [138]). Emotion detection using EmoLex identified emotions including anger, fear, anticipation, trust, surprise, sadness, joy, and disgust.

The trends of polarity were evaluated over time. This helped in interpreting the data, for example by concluding that sentiment became more intensively negative following an increase in COVID-19 media coverage or that rising emotional contagion might represent a warning on different stressors affecting psychological well-being during the outbreak [39].

The study concluded that analysing social media like Twitter is an essential part of surveillance tools to support the management of the pandemic and "its waves might actually represent a novel preventive approach to hinder emotional contagion, disseminating reliable information and nurturing trust" [39].

13.6 Providing Quality Information About Hospitals

13.6.1 The Problem

Online reviews provide information about hospitals, the service quality of physicians, other staff services, on hospital facilities and affordability. However, there are many reviews available online. Having an aggregated view would make it easier for patients to retrieve useful information. Additionally, hospital administrators would be able to compare to their hospital competitors, which might help in identifying opportunities for patient care improvement.

13.6.2 Solution Overview

In 2021, a life science research team from Mount Sinai Hospital collected more than 30,000 online customer reviews from 500 hospitals and then performed an aspect-based sentiment analysis, comparing the hospitals according to four aspects: Doctors' services, staffs' services, hospital facilities and affordability [9].

13.6.3 Methods and Procedures

The hospital reviews were collected from online websites using web scraping. After downloading and removing HTML tags, the remaining text was processed using NLP techniques. Several pre-processing tasks such as spelling correction, removal of special characters, stop words or punctuations were realised using the Python Library TextBlob. The Natural language toolkit NLTK was used for lemmatisation and negation handling. Polarity at sentence-level was conducted using SentiWordNet. The process is visualised in Fig. 13.4.

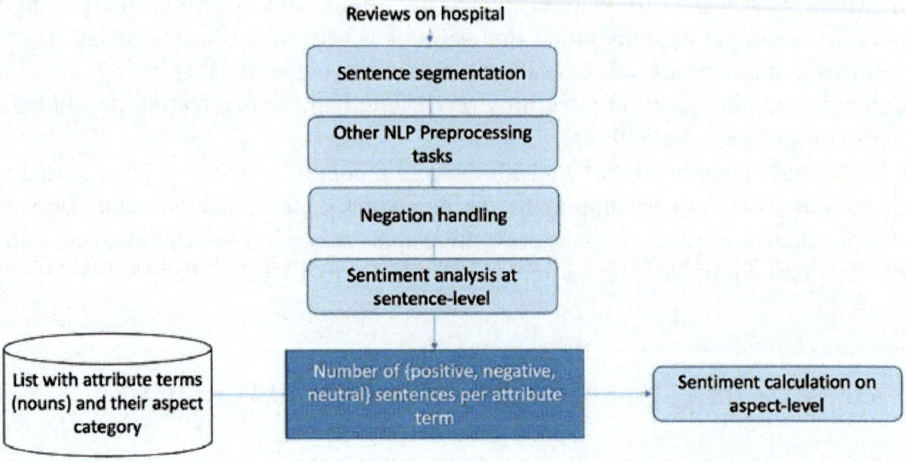

Fig. 13.4 Process of identifying polarities on quality-related aspects of hospitals

Nouns of all reviews were extracted and sorted by frequency. In a manual process, 50 nouns were selected as attributes, i.e. representing some quality-related aspects of a hospital. These attribute terms were in turn grouped into 4 categories or aspects: doctor's services, staff's services, hospital facilities, affordability (of hospital). Each sentence can contain none, one or more attribute terms. For each attribute term, the number of positive, negative and neutral sentences was counted. The rating of each aspect was calculated based on the rating of all its attribute terms by averaging the ratings. Finally, polarity for each of the four aspects was visualised per hospital for assessment by the user [9].

Part IV
Future

Chapter 14
Medical Sentiment Analysis: Quo Vadis?

14.1 SWOT Strategy

The idea of a SWOT analysis originates in strategic management research, thus providing a high practical orientation. Adapting this to sentiment analysis, we consider strengths and weaknesses as features of sentiment analysis itself, or 'internal' features. Conversely, opportunities include the economic, technical, social, political, legal, and environmental features representing the context of sentiment analysis. We thus consider opportunities to be 'external' features. Threats are, similarly, external features that may prevent further real-world implementation of medical sentiment analysis.

With this SWOT analysis, I summarise internal and external factors related to the implementation of medical sentiment analysis in practice, identify risks and issues that need solving before medical sentiment analysis can become part of the daily healthcare business and evaluate its potential for growth. Relevant questions driving the SWOT analysis are listed in Table 14.1. The following chapters will elaborate on some of the factors. The book will finish with a roadmap for future research related to medical sentiment analysis outlining the currently limiting factors that should be addressed.

14.2 Strengths

There are various applications for sentiment analysis applied to texts with medical content, which makes this technique distinctive. Sentiment analysis of medical social media data offers the opportunity of getting insights into perceptions of the public and into information demands. As a response and based on this information, public health information campaigns might be launched, or items like pharmaceuticals or medical equipment can be enhanced. For pharmaceutical companies, it is

K. Denecke, *Sentiment Analysis in the Medical Domain*,
https://doi.org/10.1007/978-3-031-30187-2_14

Table 14.1 Questions driving the SWOT analysis

	Strengths	Weaknesses
Internal features	What is unique about medical sentiment analysis? What are advantages of medical sentiment analysis? What are the biggest achievements of applying such methods? Could medical sentiment analysis already be used to significantly support the healthcare system in its tasks?	What are the disadvantages of medical sentiment analysis? Are the methods and tools sufficiently developed for the modern healthcare market? Are the results of medical sentiment analysis useful for healthcare professionals and are they accepted at all? What needs improvement in the context of medical sentiment analysis?
	Opportunities	Threats
External features	Which external changes in the context of healthcare and the overall market will bring opportunities? What are current trends supporting medical sentiment analysis? Is there any gap in the market that can be addressed by medical sentiment analysis? Can medical sentiment analysis benefit from other (health) technologies?	What are current trends preventing success of medical sentiment analysis? Which serious concerns from health professionals or other stakeholders exist that prevent the actual implementation of medical sentiment analysis? Is health technology sufficiently prepared to integrate medical sentiment analysis?

for instance a method to analyse first-hand information relevant for post-market surveillance and monitoring.

Applying sentiment analysis tools to medical social media data is already popular at least within clinical research. It was used to study community needs and perceptions of different disease communities including autism and Asperger syndrome [16, 67]. Using sentiment analysis in interactive systems to create empathetic reactions is just another step towards human-likeness of such systems. Medical sentiment analysis also offers new research possibilities: Besides understanding emotions and feelings associated with living with diseases by means of social media analysis, the impact of sentiment and emotion on behaviour change techniques could be studied. From online reviews or other textual sources, patient preferences can be determined which supports adjusting health interventions to the patient‘s needs.

An automatic processing and analysis of sentiment in clinical narratives helps to make use of so far unconsidered or hidden information captured in such documents. This helps in identifying therapy needs and provides guidance for clinical decision-making. Although not yet arrived in clinical practice, several research papers show the potentials medical sentiment analysis could have in healthcare. Research related to mortality or readmission risk prediction demonstrates that the currently almost unused resource of clinical notes can contribute to predicting risks at an earlier stage of treatment [127, 198, 210].

The ability to recognise emotions of patients may be important for health monitoring and risk prevention. As exemplified, information on the mental health status of an individual can be collected or risks for developing psychological or mental health problems can be detected. Considering sentiment and emotions systematically can add a new dimension to personalised medicine (P5 medicine) and enrich the digital exposome. The personalised, predictive, participatory, precision and preventive (P5) medicine model is an interdisciplinary and multidisciplinary approach that will make a comprehensive body of information in the management of diseases available to researchers and clinicians [19].

Medical sentiment analysis offers opportunities for digital health interventions that are increasingly developed and made available. Integrating methods of medical sentiment analysis into digital health interventions has potential to support acceptance and improve outcomes of those interventions. Interactive systems can incorporate empathy which could make their recommendations more relevant when the sentiment of the user is considered. Empathy can significantly improve medical outcomes, raise patient satisfaction, and decrease malpractice litigation [46]. The patient's perceptions and the clinician's actions, including nonverbal cues like intonation and nonverbal cues like body language, are what form the basis of the empathetic clinician-patient connection. However, there may be grounds for concern given the digitisation of healthcare services and the resulting decrease of empathy in healthcare. Equipping a digital health intervention with medical sentiment analysis functionalities to recognise patient‘s concerns and fears could address this concern since the system interaction becomes more human-like.

14.3 Weaknesses

Similar to other tasks within natural language processing, medical sentiment analysis is only able to recognise information that is in the data. The reliability of recognised information can be questioned in particular when the content of the textual sources is unreliable. Even for clinical narratives the question may arise whether the correctness or relevance of the data is sufficient or representative to have trust in the results of medical sentiment analysis. I will elaborate on this again in Chap. 16 when discussing bias and other ethical aspects. However, when accepting results of medical sentiment analysis as additional piece of information worth considering it might become useful.

Reported accuracies for sentiment analysis from the medical social web achieve in average 79.8% (maximum of 88.6 %) as reported by Zunic et al. [212]. For clinical narratives, average accuracy of the sentiment classification ranges from 71.5–88.2 % and the F1-measure lies between 50–65 %. This is well below accuracy achieved for sentiment analysis for movie reviews, which is typically larger than 90% [148]. There is still potential to improve the quality of analysis. In particular, it is still unclear how medical sentiment analysis performs on real world clinical documents. Most of the studies that are published on sentiment analysis from clinical narratives exploit the data from the i2b2 challenge or MIMIC. In this way, the methods become tuned to this writing. Applying a classifier trained on these data on other texts might lead to a loss of accuracy.

Research on medical sentiment analysis concentrated on processing texts in English. This might be due to the fact that datasets and lexical resources in other languages are rare. Limited research has been conducted in Spanish [45, 97, 158] or on tweets in multiple languages [126]. This can be seen as weakness for real-world application since transfer to other languages would require developing language-specific resources and developing methods that can handle language-specific peculiarities.

14.4 Opportunities

There are several trends in healthcare that can contribute to the opportunities of medical sentiment analysis. The availability of online tools for posting reviews and perceptions after undergoing a treatment—and their use by patients—places demands on healthcare provider in analysing this data and come up with strategies how to deal with the analysis results. Since pharmaceutical companies are legally obliged to conduct post-market surveillance, they might become a driver for medical sentiment analysis—at least from social media data. These methods provide support in analysing the huge amounts of data published online related to drugs.

The concept of lean management increased in interest in hospitals. One aspect of lean is involvement of employees in quality management and assurance. The voices of the employee and the voices of the patients are critical for quality improvement. This development contributes to the relevance of medical sentiment analysis since it allows to easily analyse, interpret and aggregate natural language feedback. The results can be used for developing quality improvement strategies.

Medical sentiment analysis allows healthcare practitioners to aggregate data from patient feedback. This allows to easier see where a practise thrives, which processes need to improve, and which capabilities are weak.

Several use cases have been described in Chap. 2 demonstrating that for example healthcare service provider can benefit from medical sentiment analysis. From a business or quality assessment perspective opportunities are related to business intelligence, reputation management and competitive analysis which become possible through medical sentiment analysis. Healthcare organisations can identify areas for strategy improvement by using medical sentiment analysis.

Solutions providing information on healthcare services for patients can be developed making use of sentiment analysis results. For example, the information from healthcare service reviews can be aggregated and visualised in a manner that is easily understandable to patients and providing them with better insights into the healthcare provider quality [9]. Developing tools like this goes along with the trend in healthcare aiming at empowering the patients and equipping them with tools to actively make decisions.

Medical sentiment analysis will allow for an improved understanding of patients. Through collecting, examining, and analysing patients' opinions, researcher and healthcare professionals will learn how patients feel about their healthcare treatment, a drug or a healthcare service. Being aware of the "patient voice" could help in adjusting healthcare services to user needs.

Another trend in healthcare that contributes to the relevance of medical sentiment analysis is the digitisation in the healthcare domain. Electronic health records become available; clinical data warehouses are installed capturing the clinical data including clinical narratives that could be analysed regarding sentiment with several use case scenarios in prediction and quality assessment.

Lifestyle medicine, i.e. the medical speciality that uses therapeutic lifestyle interventions as a primary modality to treat medical conditions, gains in interest in particular for treating chronic conditions or cancer. In this field, not only measurable objective values are of interest, but also quality of life, i.e. subjective observations. Medical sentiment analysis could support by collecting, analysing and interpreting such subjective observations making them available for lifestyle medicine.

These examples just outline a few possible opportunities that might contribute to the success of medical sentiment analysis. In particular developing use cases for medical sentiment analysis from clinical narratives is still in its beginning. Additional clinical use cases going beyond predicting the readmission risk or 30-day mortality might become of interest.

14.5 Threats

The currently missing lexical and data resources hamper the success of medical sentiment analysis. As outlined before, clinical data is difficulty to access. Once the methods for sentiment analysis become integrated into clinical decision support tools or other information systems the data would be available much easier. However, at the current stage, datasets annotated with sentiments still have to be made available in different languages and for different facets of medical sentiment. Beyond lexicons are missing and have to be developed specifically for the medical domain. This process is not yet scaleable.

In order to predict readmission risks or other clinical endpoints using medical sentiment analysis, many researchers have used unspecialised tools (such as TextBlob) on clinical data up to now without thoroughly evaluating the quality of the instrument they used. Medical sentiment analysis may not be successful if these tools are of poor quality: The following risk prediction may also be inaccurate if the medical sentiment analysis's findings are incorrect. Because of this, systems may struggle to deliver the necessary quality, limiting sentiment analysis from being applied more widely in therapeutic settings.

Another aspect that can threat the success of medical sentiment analysis is a potential misinterpretation and ethical questions that raise from an automatic analysis of emotions and sentiment of patients (probably even without letting them know). Ethical and unintended implications will be outlined in a separate section of this book (Chap. 16).

A number of linguistic phenomena of language have to be addressed in order to achieve high accuracy. In particular characteristics of clinical language and language in social media could hamper the quality of medical sentiment analysis. Some of these phenomena include complexity of clinical language and abbreviations, or sarcasm and irony in social media. A more detailed outline is given in Chap. 15.

It can be assumed that medical sentiment analysis from clinical narratives can only be successful when integrated in clinical workflows, i.e. in clinical information systems. Being part of clinical decision support systems is essential to—at the one hand—have access to the clinical data, and—on the other hand—to appropriately support in the clinical workflow.

Chapter 15
Open Challenges Related to Language

15.1 Specific Language Phenomena Hampering Sentiment Analysis

In this section, language phenomena are described that can occur in clinical narratives or medical social media texts and that may hamper medical sentiment analysis. Most of the phenomena described appear more often in clinical narratives given their length and original purpose (clinical documentation) which results in a more complex language.

15.1.1 Negations

Negations are frequently used, especially in clinical narratives. This is because clinical examinations are carried out to support or refute hypotheses. For this reason, if no evidence was discovered, results are clearly negated when they are documented. Take into account the following finding report examples:

- *Colon is unremarkable.*
- *No pathologically enlarged lymph nodes.*
- *Speech is clear with no signs of slurring.*

The author of this report clearly states what was not confirmed by the examination.

There are different possibilities for expressing negations in freetext (see Table 15.1). Adding negative prefixes to nouns, adjectives, and verbs is one technique to form negative claims. English negative prefixes include: *a–*, *dis–*, *il–*, *im–*, *in-*, *ir–*, *non–*, *un–*. To negate an English verb, the negative verbal particle *not* can be added (e.g. *"I do not like this drug")*. A negative meaning can be created by attaching a negative particle to a noun group (e.g. *"No signs of slurring"*).

K. Denecke, *Sentiment Analysis in the Medical Domain*,
https://doi.org/10.1007/978-3-031-30187-2_15

Table 15.1 The various types of negations

Negation type	Description	Example
Morphological negation	Created using negation prefixes such as *-ab, -dis, -il, -ir, -un*. The negation's scope is limited to the word with the prefix.	*irrelevant, unremarkable*
Syntactical negation	Expressed by negative verbal particles, the scope of a syntactical negation is limited by the next punctuation mark, and can be extended by a coordination particle.	*No pathologically enlarged lymph nodes.*
Double negation	The scope of the double negation is limited to the word with the negation particle inside a syntactical negation scope. Semantically no negation happens to the word.	*I can't not take my prescription.*

Another option is to add a negative meaning to a sentence by including an adverb phrase with a negative meaning (e.g. using the word "*without*").

Recognising negations expressed by words like *"not, never, can't, wasn't"* etc. and their appropriate interpretation is crucial for sentiment analysis tools since reversing the meaning of the negated term or phrases might be required. Even double negations have to be processed correctly. For instance, a computer system must comprehend that the phrase *"I can't not take my prescription"* denotes the speaker's intention to take the medication. The sentence's polarity must be changed from double negative to positive. When training a machine learning model to realise this resolution, a corpus is required that is big enough to train the algorithm and has many negation terms and examples available to get aware of all possible permutations and combinations.

In this scenario, it is also critical to correctly identify the scope of the negation as well as coordination structures (for example, *"I don't like the scent of the drug, but the taste is fine"* where the negation solely refers to the "*smell*", not the "*taste*").

A negation detection algorithm, NegEx, has been developed specifically for clinical narratives [29]. NegEx identifies the trigger terms indicating that a clinical concept is negated and determines the scope of the negation. Negspacy is a spaCy pipeline for recognising negated concepts in text [129, 188]. It bases on the NegEx algorithm. Once the negation and its scope is correctly identified, its impact on the polarity has to be adequately interpreted.

15.1.2 Valence Shifters

Adverbs such as *barely, moderately* or *slightly* shift the valence of the following term or phrase as negations do. Intensifiers such as *significantly* and *very* are modifiers that do not change the content of the following phrase they modify, but they add to the emotionality or strength, i.e. they increase the impact of a sentiment-bearing word. A de-amplifier (downtoner) reduces the impact of a sentiment-bearing word.

Sentences such as *"Indeterminate right kidney mass is most likely a renal cell carcinoma"* occur frequently in clinical narratives. They express the uncertainty of the judgement. Correct interpretation of valence shifters and the values they are referring to is crucial in the medical domain since they can express certainty and uncertainty of the judgement and have a direct impact on clinical decision making.

Modality is a semantic concept that expresses the level of confidence, permission, or obligation attached to a phrase's predicate (or topic referred to). As a result, if the predicate carries a sentiment, the sentiment of the modal and predicate together may differ from the sentiment of the predicate alone. Modality in English—to mention a few—can be achieved by:

- modal verbs (will/would, can/could, may/might, shall/should, must),
- modal adverbs (maybe, perhaps, possibly, probably),
- subordinate clauses including (wish, it can be seen as, possible, probable, chance, possibility),
- modal nouns (demand, necessity, requirement, request) or
- modal adjectives (advisable, crucial, imperative, likely, necessary, probable, possible).

This is still an open research topic since only little to no work is available on automatic analysis and interpretation of modals in clinical narratives in general and in the context of medical sentiment analysis in particular.

15.1.3 Paraphrasing, Sarcasm and Irony

Sentiment can be expressed by strong sentiment-bearing words, but also in a more subtle manner. Words with strong positive (+1) and negative (−1) polarities include "*love*" and "*hate*." These are simple to comprehend and interpret automatically. However, other phrases, like "*not too bad*," can signify "average," and as a result, they have a weaker polarity. This problem is in particular of relevance when the polarity is considered as a value on a scale (e.g. any value between 0 and 1 indicates positivity, but with varying strengths). To interpret such subtle difference appropriately, it is essential to take into account individual elements or topics instead of the entire document-level as basis for the sentiment analysis. Many parts of a statement can be examined in-depth using aspect-based sentiment analysis. However, as mentioned before, aspect-based sentiment analysis is the most challenging level of analysis and has not been often considered in medical sentiment analysis.

Additionally, in medical social media, language is often used in creative and nuanced ways, and this can make it difficult for machine learning algorithms to accurately interpret and classify the sentiment of a text. For example, irony, sarcasm, and other forms of figurative language can be difficult for an algorithm to understand and interpret correctly. In medical social media, sarcasm and irony can occur. Both styles can be difficult for medical sentiment analysis because this style of writing expresses a sentiment or opinion that is opposite or contrary to what is actually being said. A correct interpretation requires an understanding of the speaker‘s intent and the context in which the statement is being made.

Irony is a figure of language in which the intended meaning is the opposite of the literal meaning of the words used. It is often used to express a sense of humour or to make a subtle point. As exemplified, someone was just diagnosed with cancer and comments: *"Great, just what I needed, another thing to worry about"*. This statement expresses frustration or annoyance, even though parts of the phrase could be interpreted as positive. For a correct interpretation, it is necessary to understand the speaker‘s intent and recognise the ironic tone. Sarcasm is a type of irony that is often used to mock or ridicule someone or something. It is characterised by a sharp, bitter or cutting tone. Overall, the complexity and subtlety of irony and sarcasm can make it challenging for sentiment analysis algorithms to accurately detect and classify.

15.1.4 Comparative Sentences

A comparative sentence is a sentence that compares two things. The comparison is usually made using adjectives or adverbs, which describe the qualities or characteristics of the things being compared. Comparative sentences may not always provide a clear opinion, which makes them challenging to understand and interpret automatically. Relevant meanings need to be inferred. For example, a finding report claims *"the tumour is larger than a walnut"*. It compares the size of the tumour with the size of a walnut. This sentence does not mention any negative or positive emotion but rather states a relative size in terms of a common food item.

In finding reports reporting on tumour sizes, comparisons with common food items are used to clarify or visualise the tumour size: size of a pea (1 cm), a peanut (2 cm), a grape (3 cm), a walnut (4 cm), a lime (5 cm or 2 inches), an egg (6 cm), a peach (7 cm), and a grapefruit (10 cm or 4 inches). A walnut would be medium-size—so would have to be interpreted with a rather negative polarity. Beyond the fact that such comparison adds a topic which is actually "out-of-topic" (a food item in a radiological report), its interpretation in terms of positive and negative requires comprehensive knowledge. Comparative sentences can also occur in social media postings, for example to express the personal feelings or experiences in a more visual manner.

Lexicon-based approaches are not useful to interpret comparative sentences. Even bag of words models cannot handle comparisons very well. For example, the phrase "*Aspirin is better than Paracetamol*" (both are drugs that can be taken against headache), would be considered positive for both drugs Aspirin and Paracetamol when using a bag of words model because the relation between the two drugs expressed by the term *"better"* is not taken into account in the bag of words.

When a sentiment model can compare whether an entity possesses a property to a greater or lesser extent than another property, better sentiment analysis accuracy can be reached in this situation. This necessitates more than just having a corpus of words with distinct positive or negative sentiments. To solve this problem, an artificial intelligence system must analyse the relationships between entities, words, and emotions more thoroughly.

15.1.5 Coordination Structures

Connecting sentences with coordinating or subordinating clauses is frequently used in clinical narratives since it produces more effective writing and more compact information. Coordination structures join two related ideas of equal importance. Phrases can be connected by conjunctive adverbs expressing for example cause and effect (e.g. accordingly, consequently, hence, thus), contrast (e.g. instead, however, conversely), emphasis (e.g. namely, certainly, indeed). Subordination sentence structures join two related ideas of unequal importance. Consider the following example phrases:

- *Normal in size and morphology.*
- *No free fluid or free air.*
- *Perineal area assessed and found to be clear and intact, no signs of redness or irritation noted.*
- *Recommend CT scan of the abdomen and pelvis with and without contrast for further evaluation.*

The challenge for sentiment analysis is to identify and assign the correct scope when phrases are coordinated and assign the polarity accordingly. For example in the phrase *Normal in size and morphology* the term *"normal"* also qualifies the noun *"morphology"*. Resolution of coordination structures is in particular of interest when analysing sentiment on a topic- or aspect-level.

15.1.6 Word Ambiguity

Word ambiguity occurs when a word has multiple meanings or can be used in different contexts, which can lead to confusion and misunderstandings. In such cases, it is impossible to define the word's polarity in advance. It is hard to create an universal sentiment lexicon with a polarity for each word and its different meanings as the meaning of words can be highly dependent on cultural and individual differences, and can change over time as language evolves.

To clarify word ambiguities, one method is to examine the context in which a word is used to ascertain its intended meaning and sentiment. In order to do this, it may be necessary to examine the words that come before and after the ambiguous term as well as the broader subject or theme of the text. Another approach is to use part-of-speech tagging to identify the role that a word plays in a sentence, which can help to disambiguate its meaning. For example, a word that is used as a verb may have a different meaning than a word that is used as a noun.

In some cases, it may be possible to resolve word ambiguity by looking up the word in a dictionary or thesaurus and identifying its possible meanings. SentiWordNet contains polarity values for different meanings of a term. However, the challenge of recognising the correct meaning remains. Language models could address this challenge since words are represented by the context. This can involve training the algorithm on a large dataset of labelled examples, in which the meaning of each word is identified. Enough training examples for all possible meanings are required.

15.2 Evolution of Language

Language is constantly evolving, and this can present challenges for medical sentiment analysis, as the meaning and connotations of words and phrases can change over time. This can make it difficult for machine learning algorithms to accurately classify the sentiment of a text, as the underlying models may not be familiar with the latest meanings and connotations of certain words or phrases.

Another challenge is that new words and phrases are constantly being introduced in the language, and these may not be recognised by sentiment analysis algorithms that were trained on older datasets. It can lead to errors in medical sentiment classification, as the algorithm may not understand the meaning of these new words or phrases.

While dictionaries such as LIWC or SentiWordNet cover a significant portion of commonly used words, the continuous evolution of language requires fixed resources to be frequently updated in order to contain all relevant vocabulary. For example when analysing sentiment in medical social media, the usage of slang can hamper the interpretation. Slang terms appear and disappear frequently so that they are probably not included in sentiment lexicons.

For clinical narratives, organisation-specific vocabularies have to be taken into account. Depending on the culture of writing clinical reports, the language use can differ between hospitals. Lexicon-based approaches to medical sentiment analysis require continuous updates to address this; machine learning-based approaches have to be retrained from time to time to include new terms and terminology into the underlying models.

Table 15.2 Linguistic challenges and their relevance for sentiment analysis on different levels. "-" refers to less relevant, "x" relevant, "(x)" partially relevant

Challenge	Document-level	Sentence-level	Aspect-level
Paraphrasing	-	x	x
Negations	x	x	x
Comparative sentences	-	x	x
Word ambiguity	x	x	x
Valence shifters	(x)	(x)	x
Coordination structures	-	-	x
Burden of language development	x	x	x

Overall, the constantly evolving nature of language can present challenges for sentiment analysis algorithms, as it can be difficult for the algorithms to accurately interpret and classify the sentiment of texts that contain new or unfamiliar words, phrases, or figurative language. Table 15.2 shows for the described language phenomena on which level of analysis they would be of relevance.

Chapter 16
Responsible Sentiment Analysis in Healthcare

16.1 Ethical Principles Applied to Medical Sentiment Analysis

This book has demonstrated how medical sentiment analysis seeks to ascertain the emotions and sentiments stated by individuals for usage in a variety of healthcare settings. Relying healthcare decisions upon information determined automatically using sentiment analysis techniques can result in unintended consequences that, on the one hand, concern the text analysis process in general and, on the other hand, concern the potential personal repercussions of this analysis. The textual information used for sentiment analysis (i.e. the nursing note or the finding report) was produced by individuals and reflect their bias, prejudices etc. Depending on whether the results are used maliciously or for good, the follow-up processing that the embedded bias, prejudices, etc. enters has the potential to cause harm. Another aspect impacting on the consequences of sentiment analysis technology is related to the extent to which medical sentiment analysis is involved in clinical decision making, i.e. whether decisions are based on the results, are driven by the results or are made by a system. This chapter provides considerations on the various aspects related to unintended consequences of medical sentiment analysis. I structure the explanations around common moral principles.

The four principles of medical ethics developed by Beauchamp and Childress have become a common framework for ethical decisions in patient care [13]. This framework is based on four moral principles: respect for autonomy, non-maleficience and beneficience and justice (see Table 16.1). Floridi et al. added to the four moral principles an additional principle for AI-based systems which is the explicability of the underlying AI methods [62]. It integrates accountability and intelligibility and enables the other four principles (respect for autonomy, non-maleficience, beneficience, justice, see Fig. 16.1).

Respect for autonomy refers to an individual's right to make own decisions. It also implies confidentiality according to Gillon [71]. Data used for medical

K. Denecke, *Sentiment Analysis in the Medical Domain*,
https://doi.org/10.1007/978-3-031-30187-2_16

Table 16.1 Examples of ethical principles and risks of medical sentiment analysis

Ethical principle	Examples of risk	Examples of mitigation
Respect for autonomy	Patients are not asked about how their (social media) data is used and which healthcare measurements are taken upon analysis results	Patient education: provide information about how the algorithms work, what they are being used for, which data will be used and the potential benefits and risks associated with their use
Non-maleficience	Datasets are re-purposed, have potential for de-identified health data to be used in ways that harm individuals	Prohibit sharing of data with third parties
Beneficience	Results of medical sentiment analysis are used to serve non-medical purposes or to manipulate individuals	Prohibit sharing of personal health data, even medical social media data, careful design of solutions, approval of health authorities (FDA or similar organisations)
Justice	Sentiment analysis algorithm misinterprets consistently sentiments of a ethnically minority group leading to unfair clinical decisions	Careful assembling of the training data, and assessment of the results by humans

sentiment analysis is normally collected from data sources even without awareness of the individuals. It is used for public health research [187] or for calculating a digital exposome using the social media content to profile an individual's mental health status. In this way, individuals whose data is used in such way are stealed from deciding actively in favour or against the data usage. Section 16.2 outlines aspects related to respect for autonomy.

The two ethical principles beneficience (acting for the welfare of an individual) and non-maleficience (doing no harm to an individual) have to be considered together [183]. These principles raise the question of responsibility and accountability: when a sentiment analysis algorithm fails in detecting the suicide risk, who is accountable for the mistake? Additionally, there is a potential for the misuse of emotion analysis. The results of emotion analysis could be used to manipulate or exploit people. They could be used to violate people's privacy, for example by monitoring their emotional states without their knowledge or consent. Section 16.3 outlines thoughts on this topic. The ethical principles of beneficence and non-maleficence are relevant in the context of medical sentiment analysis because they concern the ways in which the algorithms are used and the impact they have on patients. It is important to ensure that sentiment analysis algorithms are used in ways that are ethical and that promote the well-being of patients.

Justice concerns the idea of fairness in healthcare delivery, i.e. all patients should be treated equally and should have equitable access to healthcare resources [183]. When applying machine learning algorithms to patient data for realising medical sentiment analysis, multiple instances of biases can be induced which might impact

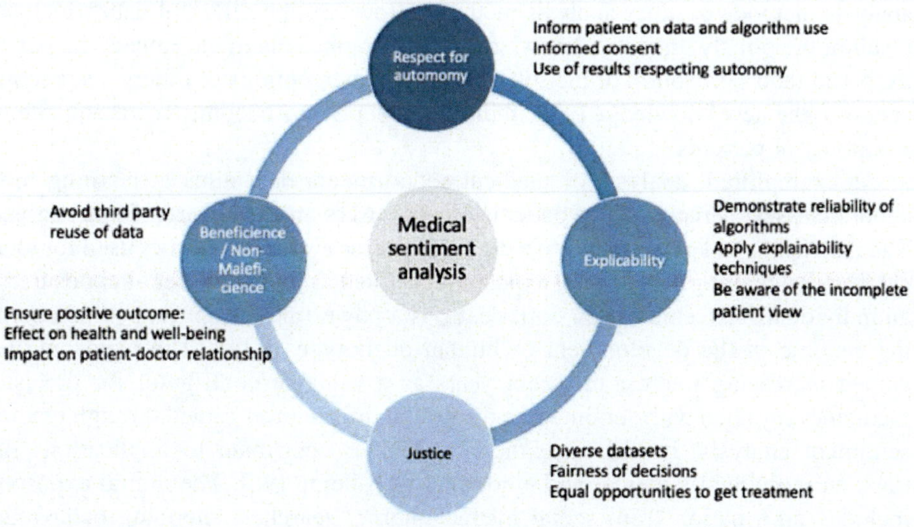

Fig. 16.1 Ethical principles and related aspects to consider within medical sentiment analysis grouped by the four moral principles (respect for autonomy, beneficience/non-maleficience, Justice) and a fifth principle added as relevant for AI systems

on the clinical decision making and might threaten the principle of justice. Details are provided in Sect. 16.4.

Finally, there is the issue of transparency and explicability. It is important that algorithms and methods used for sentiment and emotion analysis are transparent and explainable, so that the results can be understood and evaluated by the people who are being affected by them or making decisions based on the results. More details on transparent algorithms, explainability and its relation to trust are described in Sect. 16.5 and Chap. 17.

Topics that are raised in the following are also discussed in the context of biobanking, medical artificial intelligence in general, or data ethics. It is out of scope of this book to comprehensively discuss relevant aspects. The objective of the following sections is to raise awareness and trigger reflections.

16.2 Respect for Autonomy

Respect for autonomy refers to the ethical principle of respecting individuals' right to make decisions for themselves and to act independently. In the context of healthcare, this principle is relevant because patients have the right to make decisions about their own healthcare and treatment; and healthcare professionals have a responsibility to respect and support these decisions. The amount of data available on a person increases due to the digitisation. Persons even share data on their own for example in social media. Analysing this data by medical sentiment analysis methods or other analysis methods allows to link different data which can result in previously unknown knowledge on a person. This might impact the person itself and their perception of the self, but also the perceptions of others that become access to the new knowledge [92]. In this context privacy becomes a prerequisite for autonomy of patients.

As exemplified, analysis of medical social media data aims at learning more about diseases, perceptions of patients etc. but users are not aware of this analysis. The data could be aggregated into a digital exposome which is further used for clinical decision making. The digital exposome, defined as the whole set of exposures of an individual from conception until death, is a powerful concept that complements the genome in the development of human phenotypes [200]. The exposome has gained increasing interest in recent years as a valuable contributor for precision medicine; enriched with sentiment and emotion information gained through medical sentiment analysis, it will have the potential to contribute to applications that track an individual‘s mental and emotional well-being [96]. The digital exposome includes information from social media, internet searches, shopping behaviours, and other types of digital activity. The classic idea of the exposome, which refers to the collection of environmental exposures that a person encounters during their lifetime, is considered as a supplement by those who study the digital exposome. The digital exposome comprises exposures connected to digital technology and the online environment, whereas the classic exposome includes exposures related to air pollution, diet, and physical exercise. The digital exposome is of interest to researchers and healthcare professionals because it can provide insights into an individual’s behaviours, preferences, and exposures to digital content, which may be relevant to their health and well-being. By analysing the digital exposome, it may be possible to identify patterns and trends that can help to inform the development of interventions or policies that promote health and prevent disease.

Results from medical sentiment analysis can inform the digital exposome with information on emotions and sentiments. Overall, a patient has a right to get informed on all aspects concerning their life and health. However, being aware of how algorithms judge an individual‘s emotions and sentiments might have an impact on the person‘s sense of self which in turn can impact on their individual decision making. Interpretation of the data might be difficult for patients. In this context it is important to ensure that patient‘s maintain their autonomy on their data and related consequences. This could involve providing information about how the algorithms work, what they are being used for, which data will be used and the potential benefits and risks associated with their use.

An aspect related to respect for autonomy in the context of medical sentiment analysis is to ensure that patients are aware of and have the opportunity to give informed consent to the use of medical sentiment analysis algorithms in their care and to the analysis of their data using these methods. Informed consent is the process of a patient being informed about the procedures and risks associated with any medical care prior to giving their approval. It is a fundamental part of healthcare and an important part of patient autonomy. Informed consent is required before any medical procedure is applied, allowing a patient to make an informed decision about their care. In the context of biobanking, a new type of consent has been established given the situation that the patient will not know which analyses will be conducted on their data and which conclusions can be drawn in future [82]. Discussions on something similar for artificial intelligence-based systems started already [8]. Application of medical sentiment analysis methods often results in retrospective data mining for purposes not anticipated when patients consented to allow their data to be used. This means similar discussions related to informed consent to medical sentiment analysis still have to be conducted.

Additionally, predicting information using clinical notes might reveal information patients were not willing to disclose (e.g. likelihood of adherence to the therapy, frequency of engagement in smoking). Predicting such information without patient consent could be interpreted as privacy violation [175] and is not respecting the autonomy of the patient to decide for disclosing information.

Besides consenting to the use of data another important aspect is to ensure that the results of sentiment analysis are used in a way that respects the autonomy of the patient. This could involve using the results to inform discussions between patients and healthcare professionals, rather than making decisions on behalf of the patient relying upon the sentiment analysis results. In the latter case, medical sentiment analysis would weaken the role of the patient and criticisms could be raised whether the decision making of a patient gets really supported or undermined. In 2019, Facebook developed a Suicide Algorithm[1] intended to monitor online behaviour and alert local law enforcement when a suicide risk was detected. The algorithm seriously harms patient's autonomy and ignores confidentiality and consent.

16.3 Beneficience and Non-maleficience

Beneficence refers to the ethical principle of acting in the best interests of the patient, and it requires healthcare professionals to do good and avoid harm. Consider sentiment analysis algorithms that could be used to identify patients who are at risk of developing mental health problems, so that healthcare professionals can intervene and provide the necessary support. This would be an example of beneficence, as it would involve acting in the best interests of the patient by identifying and addressing potential health issues. At the same time the question arises how to define a health risk. Who defines the risks and are the risks justifying the collection and processing of the data?

The ethical principle of not harming the patients or working against their best interests is known as non-maleficence. In the context of sentiment analysis, it would be important to ensure that the results generated by the algorithms are not causing

[1] https://www.businessinsider.co.za/facebook-is-using-ai-to-try-to-predict-if-youre-suicidal-2018-12.

harm or support acting against the best interests of the patients. For example, the principle of non-maleficience would be harmed when based on sentiment analysis results decisions are made that are not in the best interests of patients or manipulate decision makers. In the context of medical sentiment analysis, the principle of non-maleficience can be hurt when data gained through the analysis is misused for unauthorised purposes which could create harm in a person.

An algorithm or IT system being of benefit for patients entails protecting and advancing their wellness as well as their interests [15]. Well-being can concern: (1) objective functioning/health and (2) the patient's view of their own good. Questions going along with this include: What is the potential clinical utility of a system using medical sentiment analysis? Does the prediction of a medical event based on medical sentiment analysis lead to clinical benefits? E.g. when predicting the readmission risk, are there methods or strategies available that would help to avoid readmission? Medical sentiment analysis is of benefit for a patient when the system has a positive outcome on the patient‘s health and well-being. Risk prediction systems considering results from medical sentiment analysis can help with early risk prevention when their results are used to take steps to lower the risk at an early stage of the treatment process. The question remains whether healthcare professionals would be able to address the risks appropriately once the sentiment analysis-based system recognises an increased risk. What can be done when a risk is predicted?

From a patient‘s perspective, medical sentiment analysis can contribute to improved access to information. Consider the platform that was introduced in Sect. 13.6 that aggregates quality aspects from healthcare provider to support decision making of patients. The pure amount of information of hospital quality could not be accessed by patients (or only with a lot of effort) but the platform allows to get this information. In such case, medical sentiment analysis would be of benefit at a first instance (and when the patient is able to act accordingly, also in a second instant).

Related to this are concerns and criticism that making predictions or classifying patients regarding their mental health issues, suicide risk or similar aspects based on EHR data can have the effect of creating a distance to the patient: analysing indirect observations of patients written by health professionals might ignore the patient voice. This might lead to potential increases in stigma, and privacy violations [175]. The question arises how to safeguard patient privacy.

Analysing textual data with medical sentiment analysis methods generates also risks for privacy and security. As exemplified, once collected, data can be almost infinitely repurposed, re-analysed and shared or even combined with other datasets. This may result in additional unintended consequences, and privacy as well as security can be harmed.

Machine learning-based systems to sentiment analysis involve the access to large quantities of data regarding patients and healthy citizens. This makes demands regarding the ownership of data, informed consent and good data sharing practices. Recent regulatory initiatives such as the European Union's General Data Protection Regulation (GDPR) or the Health Insurance Portability and Accountability Act (HIPAA) raised awareness on security in IT systems. Data security relates to the protection of data against unauthorised access or to avoid its theft or misuse [104]. These initiatives created a minimal set of expectations for data privacy and the associated data security. Both regulations provide a set of guidelines stipulating how personally identifiable data or information should be maintained by healthcare applications and healthcare insurance industries to protect them from fraud and theft.

The GDPR is demanding for purpose limitation, data minimisation, storage limitation and transparency, which is conflicting with practices of AI: data has to be reused for learning; it is impossible to identify all future purposes or data usages at the time of data collection; algorithms are often black boxes hampering transparency [125]. Also according to GDPR, mechanisms have to be in place so users may request that all their private data is deleted. However in practice, it is still unclear what level of control individuals have over the data collected on them and re-used in machine learning models and which—probably unintended—consequences this could have. A regulatory framework and corresponding technical realisations would be required for example to remove individual's data from trained models.

16.4 Justice

There are multiple factors that impact on health and well-being as well as on outcome of treatments. These include social and economic factors (e.g. income, education, culture), physical environments (e.g. food, employment, working conditions) as well as individual characteristics and behaviours (e.g. sex and gender, genetics, personal behaviour, nutrition) [35]. However, the current implementations of medical sentiment analysis demonstrate potential biases of algorithms and data sets towards such factors and resulting subgroups of the population. We have seen applications of medical sentiment analysis that impact on clinical decision making or on measurements taken. Such decisions can become unfair when the underlying medical sentiment analysis algorithms or datasets fortify biases.

Desirable and undesirable bias can be distinguished. The careful implementation of medical sentiment analysis algorithms could also help to consider bias such as sex and gender differences to achieve a more effective treatment for an individual patient. This can be considered a desirable bias.

Problematic is undesirable bias that exhibits unnecessary discrimination of subgroups [35]. Machine learning-based algorithms to medical sentiment analysis are limited by the quality of the data on which the algorithms are trained. Thus, sources of undesirable bias include not representative datasets, i.e. datasets that do not include relevant population groups (e.g. leaving minorities out) or datasets that are not generalisable. This may for instance be due to the data collection process or composition of the dataset. We recognised in Part II that clinical datasets for training medical sentiment analysis models are rare. However, to obtain models that are generalisable, data from multiple sources, on diverse people, and from a sufficient number of people would be needed in a sufficient manner [136]. If medical sentiment analysis algorithms use data that are generated through a biased process, then the output may be similarly biased.

Since they are trained on human-generated data, sentiment and emotion analysis methods can potentially reinforce and amplify inappropriate human biases. For instance, word embeddings could be learned from a biased dataset [30]. Undesirable biases can be introduced in datasets through documented human stereotypes. Recent research has demonstrated that the vast majority of sentiment and emotion analysis machine learning systems consistently assigns varying emotion ratings to statements involving various races and genders [25]). These biases frequently span stereotyped boundaries; for instance, statements about women are frequently perceived as being more emotional (more happy or sad) than phrases about men or medical doctors are connected more frequently to male pronouns than female pronouns [25].

Another challenge for bias and induced inequity is the selection of the data. When applying sentiment analysis to medical social media data, our models learn from data where individuals have chosen to self-disclose or act on their difficulties. In contrast, we are missing all individuals who are not describing their emotions and feelings online. If healthcare is relying upon data models learned from the "wrong" or incomplete data, a large cohort of patients will be omitted from care.

For these reasons greater attention has to be placed on how sentiment and emotion analysis resources are trained and used (training data, lexicons, algorithms, etc.). and their role in creating fair emotion or sentiment-based systems. Mohammad described various ethical considerations in the use of word–emotion association lexicons [135]. One aspect mentioned is that sentiment lexicons basically capture implicit emotions , i.e. words are associated with sentiment or emotions which does not mean that they really mean the emotion. Diverse socio-cultural groups have different perspectives on the meaning of words; when one particular perspective is consolidated in a lexicon, it becomes reinforced and may result in misleading impressions.

Social media was used during the COVID-19 pandemic to identify information needs and public opinions on the public health strategies. But, whose needs are retrieved through this channel? And who will benefit from the measurements derived from this analysis? There might be a risk that only a subset of the population can be covered. As long as health authorities are aware of this and also distribute measurements or run information campaigns through different channels, fairness of healthcare delivery can be achieved.

16.5 Explicability and Trust

Trust plays a central role in the healthcare domain [108]. The patient-doctor relationship is based on trust, openness, and mutual respect. Doctors need to trust that their patients are providing honest information about their symptoms and medical history in order to best diagnose and treat their condition. Patients need to trust that their doctor is providing them with accurate information and providing them with the best course of treatment for their condition. When technology such as medical sentiment analysis enters these dynamics, an additional technology-user relationship impacts on trust.

Trust is defined as a "firm belief in the reliability, truth, ability, or strength of someone or something" [201]. In the context of AI, La Rosa and Danks provide a contrasting definition. They distinguish two types of trust: trust can be grounded in reliability (the behaviour of the trustee is predictable) and trust can be grounded in an understanding of mechanisms (the trustor can generalise her knowledge to predict the trustee's behaviours and intentions; explicability is guaranteed) [108]. From these types of trust, we can derive that in order to build trust in medical sentiment analysis, these systems have to prove they are reliable and patients as well as health professionals have to understand the underlying mechanisms (see Chap. 17).

Reliability can among other things concern the data, its processing and storage by sentiment analysis algorithms. To avoid that patients and health professionals are neglective against medical sentiment analysis systems it has to be made obvious how the data will be used and how the algorithms are working. The term "explicability" describes how well humans can comprehend and justify the choices and forecasts produced by a machine learning model. This is a crucial factor to take into account because it can help to ensure that the model is transparent, responsible, and capable of producing decisions that can be trusted. Explicability is crucial in the healthcare domain, where poor or biased judgement can have serious repercussions.

Onora O'Neill's arguments in favour of transparency since it can help to create trust between individuals and organisations [153] which can be transferred also to technology. Transparency of medical sentiment analysis allows individuals to clearly see how algorithms work, which data is used, allowing them to make more informed decisions and form more reliable judgements about the results. This makes demands towards the medical sentiment analysis algorithms regarding explicability and interpretability, and also raises questions regarding accountability for their results and related actions. Onora O'Neill argues that transparency can add to the ways in which the public can be deceived because it is often possible to manipulate data or interpretations of data to support one's own agenda. Transparency can also be used to deliberately mislead. For example, figures or data that are presented in a selective or one-sided manner can create a distorted view of reality, which can ultimately lead to a lack of trust between individuals and systems based upon medical sentiment analysis.

The question arises which data is trustworthy being aware that we will never have a complete view on a patient‘s health. Datasets in medicine are naturally imperfect (due to noise, errors in documentation, incompleteness, differences in documentation granularities, etc.). For this reason it is impossible to develop machine learning models and sentiment analysis algorithms without any errors. Reliability of algorithms and systems can be demonstrated by successful outcomes and supportive functionalities. Additionally, trust in medical technology is closely related to its anticipated utility [206]. Trust will suffer when the current clinical workflow is interrupted or hampered. Thus, interoperability and integration of medical sentiment analysis methods with existing health IT systems is important.

A first step toward achieving trust in machine learning-based technologies (including medical sentiment analysis methods relying upon machine learning) was made by the EU commission who established guidelines for trustworthy AI in healthcare. According to the guideline published in 2019 [177], trustworthy AI should be:

- lawful—respecting all applicable laws and regulations,
- ethical—respecting ethical principles and values,
- robust—both from a technical perspective while taking into account its social environment.

As technical methods for trustworthy AI, the EU commission suggests among other things explanation methods, as well as methods for testing and validating. Among the non-technical methods are certification, standardisation, education and awareness to foster an ethical mindset [177]. Other suggestions to build trust in AI applications include: (1) disclosing implementation details of AI algorithms, the nature of training sets and shortcomings of the AI systems. (2) Develop interpretable machine learning models. (3) Patient education and providing more transparency into machine learning models.

A multitude of research on medical sentiment analysis considered social media data. This requires scraping data from the web. It is still debatable whether discussion forums are public domain and their data can be collected for research purposes [79]. Social media forum members might be unaware that their postings are subject to be monitored. It is suggested to at least resist on collecting identifiable information such as user name or demographic data when conducting a medical social media analysis. However, there is still no consensus about the ethical aspects of this type of research [79]. Another question is whether, how and to what extent such data should be used when interacting with patients.

16.6 Concluding Remarks

This chapter raised several aspects related to the unintended consequences of medical sentiment analysis and its use for healthcare research purposes. Similar discussions are already conducted in the context of AI use in healthcare and biobanking. A peculiarity of analysing sentiment is that text, in particular patient-generated content, can contain unconscious behaviours and emotional reactions which provides even more risks for the individual when the data is misinterpreted or misused or emotional profiles are generated. As long as the algorithms' quality is not significantly developed there is a high risk of systematic bias and discrimination.

Chapter 17
Explainable Sentiment Analysis

17.1 Definition and Need for XAI

We have observed that deep learning and machine learning models have been investigated and recommended in medical sentiment analysis. The fundamental characteristics and data representations that a model employs to categorise into sentiment categories may, however, be understood only to a limited extent. There are transparent models such as tree-based models, k-nearest neighbour or regression models whose decision processes are transparent.

However, the majority of machine learning models including SVM or neural networks do not explain how or why decisions are made. In other words, these black-box algorithms are opaque and difficult to understand. In particular in the medical domain, black-box systems whose decision-making process are not transparent can provide a risk for patient safety [211]. In order to trust a sentiment analysis-based decision support system, a physician (1) has to be able to understand the predictions (in terms of being aware of how the predictions were made, which data contributed to the decision and how), (2) has to be sure that the decision will not pose a risk for patient safety, (3) is sure that decisions are ethical, (4) has a proof that the system's results are reliable and accurate and that sensitive patient data is protected.

Moreover, the need for explanatory systems is required by regulations like the General Data Protection Regulation (GDPR). Besides the regulatory need for explanations, it might be useful for clinicians to uncover manifestations and patterns that led to data-based decisions that otherwise would remain unrecognised.

An emerging area of machine learning called explainable artificial intelligence (XAI) focuses on how artificial intelligence systems make judgements. It refers to methodologies and procedures that result in answers that are understandable by humans. XAI helps in understanding decisions and enables traceability of actions taken. It has the potential to increase human comprehension of AI made decisions, assess the legitimacy of computer-based decisions, foster trust, and lessen bias.

K. Denecke, *Sentiment Analysis in the Medical Domain*,
https://doi.org/10.1007/978-3-031-30187-2_17

XAI pursues several goals including reliability, trust, fairness, privacy, causality, transparency and usability [59]. Transparency of medical sentiment analysis models and algorithms is needed by physicians to understand the model's decisions and to be able to decide on their reliability when it comes to decisions that are critical to patient safety. Privacy indicates whether external agents can access the original data. In healthcare contexts, it is crucial to carefully consider data privacy and it should not be harmed by AI technologies. Causality concerns the relations between model variables. Studying causality is useful when analysing large amounts of health-related data since it can provide insights into relations and dependencies that otherwise would remain unconsidered. Assessing whether a machine learning model makes fair decisions is crucial to avoid bias and ethical discrimination. Trust reflects the confidence in a model's ability to perform in the face of a challenge. Usability describes how effectively and safely a technology can communicate with a user.

17.2 Explainable AI Methods

There are several methods available that can be used to explain AI models when generated from text-related features, including feature importance, sensitivity analysis and local-interpretable model-agnostic explanations (LIME). A comprehensive overview on the various methods is provided by Holzinger et al. [88]. There are different categories of explainability: Explanation can be achieved by simplification, by feature relevance explanation, by local explanation or visual explanation [14]. Feature relevance estimation provides information about how a model uses certain features or variables. Most prominent methods are gradient-based approaches. Feature relevance estimation can help to identify which features are most important for the model and how they contribute to the model's output [83]. Sensitivity analysis can support in evaluating how sensitive a model's predictions are to changes to the input data [168]. The underlying premise is that the output will be most sensitive to the input properties that are most relevant to it. This can help in determining the variables that affect a model's predictions the most. Further, it is helpful to detect potential errors or biases in the model.

LIME is a local explainability method that can be used to provide human-understandable explanations for the predictions made by a model [164]. It explains a prediction of a machine learning model for a query point by finding identifying significant predictors and building a straightforward, interpretable model. This can be helpful for explaining why a model made a specific prediction and can raise the model's level of transparency and trust. The main idea underlying LIME is that it is far simpler to approximate a black-box model locally (in the neighbourhood of the prediction we want to explain) by a simple model than it is to attempt to approximate it globally.

The information gained from an XAI method depends on the method used since the methods produce different types of output. Text-based explanation methods generate human-readable explanations. Additionally, feature statistics and feature summaries can be visualised. Argument-based explanation methods outline the features in a way to help humans in understanding the relevance of the features in making a decision [209].

17.3 Applications of XAI to Medical Sentiment Analysis

Turcan et al. suggested emotion-infused models for psychological stress detection [191]. To learn more about their trained classification models, they used LIME and identified the meaningful words that were learned by their BERT model to make the predictions. Specifically, they analysed the unigrams of the models using LIME and then applied the word lists from LIWC's psychological categories to study the types of words the classifier used to decide for one of the classes stress or non-stress.

Uban et al. applied a variety of explainability strategies to better understand the behaviour of their trained models [192]. They used deep learning to learn linguistic characteristics of mental disorders and developed a method for using social media data to early predict mental problems. To gain insights into the behaviour of their trained models, they used different explainability techniques including attention weight analysis, ablation experiments and analysis of interpretable features. An ablation study typically refers to removing some features of the model or algorithm, and seeing how that affects the model's performance. An attention weight indicates how much a particular word will be weighted when computing the next representation for the current word [36]. By using attention mechanisms, it is possible to objectively examine the behaviour of the model and confirm that it has correctly detected the links between the tokens.

Not much work has been done related to XAI in medical sentiment analysis. A reason might be that so far only few research developed machine learning models that require explanations (e.g. neural networks) and that the work is still experimental. When more clinical use cases are addressed by medical sentiment analysis researcher, I expect an increased need for explainability methods.

Chapter 18
The Future of Medical Sentiment Analysis

18.1 Current Research Gaps in Medical Sentiment Analysis

This book provided an overview on the current state-of-the art in medical sentiment analysis. Depending on the data source under consideration, i.e. clinical narratives, social media data or conversation protocols, the approaches differ, their quality of results varies and a different amount of research is yet available. I described several use cases demonstrating the potential applications of medical sentiment analysis. It is an active research field; however, several research gaps still exist, especially for analysing clinical narratives. Some limitations include:

- Limited annotated datasets: There is a lack of large, diverse, and annotated datasets for medical sentiment analysis, which makes it difficult to train and evaluate machine learning models, in particular data-hungry algorithms such as artificial neural networks.
- Domain-specific challenges: Particularly processing clinical narratives can be complex due to the language use with domain-specific terms, abbreviations, and jargon. Off-the-shelf tools are often insufficient especially when analysing clinical narratives. Research has to develop models and tools including lexicons that can effectively handle these challenges.
- Multilingual analysis: In particular when analysing medical social media data, data in different languages has to be processed. There is still a need for sentiment analysis models that can handle medical text data in multiple languages.
- Explainability and interpretability: In the medical domain, it is important to be able to understand and explain the reasoning behind a model's predictions, in particular when clinical decision making is based on the results of medical sentiment analysis. Developing models that have a high level of explainability and interpretability is an important research gap as well as applying and testing explainability methods to make trained models interpretable. Corresponding methods for achieving explainability have been presented in Chap. 17.

K. Denecke, *Sentiment Analysis in the Medical Domain*,
https://doi.org/10.1007/978-3-031-30187-2_18

- Integration with clinical decision support systems: There is an opportunity to integrate sentiment analysis models into clinical decision support systems to aid in diagnosis and treatment planning by predicting risk factors or outcomes using medical sentiment analysis results. Research is needed to understand how to effectively integrate medical sentiment analysis into the clinical workflow and how to integrate the models into clinical decision support systems.
- Patient privacy and security: When working with patient data, it is important to ensure that privacy and security are maintained. Research is needed to understand how to protect patient privacy and secure sensitive data when using sentiment analysis models. Security does not only include data security, but concerns also how to ensure patient safety and to maintain patient's autonomy.

From these research gaps, I derive five future directions for follow up research in medical sentiment analysis (see Fig. 18.1). They include working towards domain-specific resources, i.e. lexicons and datasets, testing state-of-the art machine learning methods to increase accuracy, considering methods for achieving explainability and interpretability of machine learning models and finally, demonstrate clinical benefits of applying medical sentiment analysis methods for healthcare purposes. I will provide some details on these steps in the next sections.

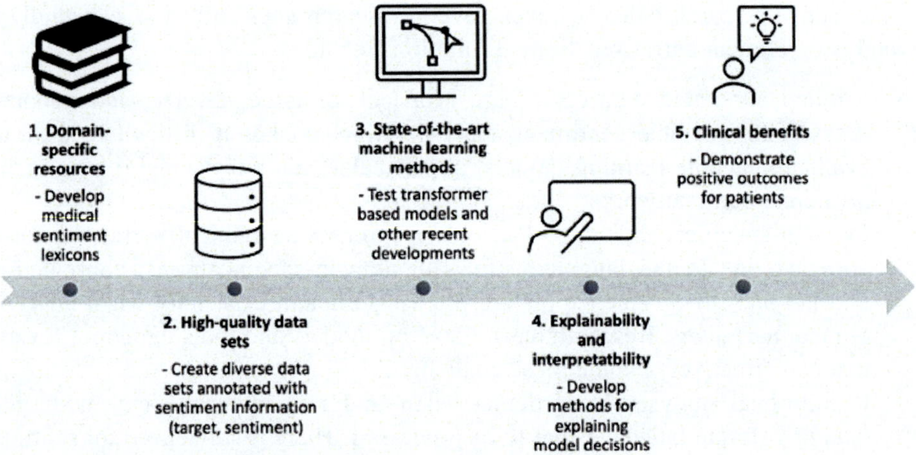

Fig. 18.1 Future directions of medical sentiment analysis

18.2 Towards Domain-Specific Resources: Lexicons and Datasets

There are several options to address the problem of unavailability of annotated datasets for medical sentiment analysis. One option is to manually annotate a dataset using human annotators, i.e. domain experts will have to label a set of medical text data regarding sentiment or emotions. This is time-consuming and resource-intensive, but it can yield high-quality annotated data. For human annotation, it is crucial to clearly define the medical sentiment under consideration, since the definition might differ depending on the medical condition under consideration (see Chap. 1).

Another option is to use transfer learning, which involves training a model on a large, general-purpose dataset and then fine-tuning it on a smaller, domain-specific dataset. Creating an annotated dataset with transfer learning can help reduce the amount of (manually) annotated data needed for training. Weak supervision techniques allow to use large amounts of unannotated or partially annotated data to train a machine learning model. For example, a rule-based classifier could automatically label a large dataset, which could then be used to train a machine learning model. We have seen that there are some annotated datasets available for medical sentiment analysis, such as those derived from the i2b2 dataset or the MIMIC dataset [53]. While these datasets may not be ideal for every research problem in medical sentiment analysis, they can offer a useful starting point for example to label automatically another dataset using a machine learning model trained on an i2b2 dataset. Equally important is to generate diverse multilingual datasets.

A community effort could also help creating and sharing a large, anonymised dataset which would support in benchmarking existing methods and could help in exploring new approaches. In collaborations with healthcare organisations access to data can be gained. The same dataset might be of interest for different research questions. A healthcare organisation can use the annotated data for their own purposes, and the researchers can use it for their sentiment analysis research. However, data privacy aspects may prevent from getting such dataset available for other researchers.

Some researchers tried already to generate patient data synthetically. Synthea is an open-source, synthetic patient generator that models the medical history of synthetic patients [194]. The aim is to provide high-quality, synthetic, realistic but not real, patient data and associated health records covering every aspect of healthcare. The resulting data is free from privacy and security restrictions. However, Synthea is not generating clinical narratives. Text generation methods such as GPT-2 have been applied to create clinical narratives [111]. Generative Pre-trained Transformer 2 (GPT-2) or its successor Generative Pre-trained Transformer 3 (GPT-3) is a language model that uses deep learning to generate text similar to some written by humans. Given an initial text as prompt, it will produce text that continues the prompt. The GPT architecture implements a deep neural network, specifically a transformer model which uses attention.

When synthetic data is used, this might not reflect the reality of clinical narratives. As exemplified, I generated a nursing note using ChatGPT (see Table 18.1). Even though some typical characteristics can be recognised (e.g. list of short phrases, use of negations, some complete sentences, use of medical terminology), real-world texts might be more diverse in terms of spelling errors or abbreviations. Another aspect to be considered when using synthetically generated clinical narratives is to ensure that the data does not amplify human bias and is balanced in terms of gender and diversity.

Sentiment lexicons used for medical sentiment analysis are basically not domain-specific. It has already been demonstrated in 2015 that general-domain sentiment lexicons are not well suited for medical sentiment analysis, since terms used in an objective manner in clinical narratives are associated with a polarity [49]. There exist two domain-specific lexicons (SentiHealth, WordNet for Medical Events) which, however, were not yet used frequently for medical sentiment analysis. General domain sentiment analysis lexicons are prevalent to realise medical sentiment analysis. Due to a more objective style of writing especially in clinical narratives,

Table 18.1 Nursing note generated by ChatGPT (https://chat.openai.com/) using the request: "Generate a progress note written by a nurse for a female person after hip transplant on the second day after surgery"

Progress note
The patient is recovering well following hip transplant surgery on Day 1. Vital signs are stable and within normal range. The patient reports minimal pain, which is currently being managed with oral pain medication.
The patient is able to move the hip with assistance and is performing range of motion exercises as instructed. She is able to ambulate with assistance and a walker. The patient is tolerating oral intake and is receiving adequate nutrition. She is able to perform deep breathing and coughing exercises to clear the lungs.
The patient is receiving physical therapy as ordered and is making progress in her mobility. The urinary catheter has been removed and the patient is able to empty her bladder independently. She is compliant with her treatment plan and able to follow instructions.
The incision site is clean and dry, with no signs of infection. The patient is able to rest comfortably and is sleeping well.
Overall, the patient is making good progress in her recovery and is on track to meet her rehabilitation goals.
Plan
– Continue to manage pain with oral medication as needed.
– Encourage the patient to ambulate with assistance and use a walker as tolerated.
– Encourage deep breathing and coughing exercises.
– Administer physical therapy as ordered.
– Monitor vital signs and incision for any changes.
– Encourage the patient to continue to follow her treatment plan and take medications as prescribed.

the conventional sentiment lexicons need to be adapted to deal with the specific characteristics of clinical narratives.

Even the meanings of terms can be different when used in clinical contexts. Consider the term *negative* in the phrase *"The COVID-19 test was negative."*. This actually has to be interpreted as something positive, since the person seems to be not infected by the virus. Denecke and Deng recognised that the context matters for correctly interpreting the medical sentiment [49]. Context can be learned from training material. Word embedding or document embedding text representations could realise this. But also a domain-specific lexicon based on a medical vocabulary such as the UMLS could be developed. In such lexicon, polarity values could be assigned to UMLS concepts.

18.3 Addressing Domain-Specific Challenges and Increasing Accuracy

There are several options to address the domain-specific challenges. First of all, research has to be conducted to find technical solutions to the language challenges described before to ensure a correct interpretation of detected sentiments (e.g. analysis of coordinated structures, negation processing). Domain-specific dictionaries and lexicons could support in adapting the machine learning models and help understanding medical terminology and jargon. Furthermore, incorporating domain knowledge into a machine learning model could help in better understanding the context and meaning of medical text. This could be realised by designing custom features or using domain-specific embeddings.

Methods for processing texts in different languages have to be developed. Even more relevant, research on aspect-based medical sentiment analysis has to be conducted since solutions would allow for a more fine-grained analysis of expressed sentiments which might be important for clinical use cases.

Research in medical sentiment analysis focuses so far on processing textual data. However, there are a range of data sources from which sentiment analysis models could benefit. These include data from wearable devices (e.g. physiological data such as heart rate or skin conductance), and mobile health apps that provide sleep patterns or geospatial movement data. In this way, a more complete digital exposome could be calculated.

In particular when considering specific medical conditions, a domain adaptation of the general sentiment definition has to be made. Disease-specific risks and their sentiment have to be defined similar as Holderness et al. did for the domain of psychiatric disorders [86]. Deng et al. considered context objects and their impact on the sentiment [53]. Other use cases may require a definition of sentiment that is covering presence, certainty or severity of symptoms as risk factors for developing a disease. It still has to be assessed when a domain-specific definition of medical sentiment is required.

The use and usefulness of considering biomedical vocabulary not only for health mention classification or topic analysis, but also within the sentiment analysis process, still has to be assessed.

Given that existing approaches to medical sentiment analysis has been most frequently conducted on i2b2 or MIMIC datasets, their performance still has to be demonstrated on real world data sets which is related to the generation of diverse annotated datasets. There is a need for more research on cross-cultural sentiment analysis. Medical sentiment analysis technologies must be trained on diverse patient datasets and must be rigorously evaluated for the various forms of bias [183].

Attention mechanism (self attention [113]) and gated multiplication (Gated CNN [203]) are increasingly tested for sentiment analysis in the open domain. However, those newly emerged methods have not yet been evaluated with data from the medical domain. Further, representation learning could be evaluated for realising medical sentiment analysis.

For the conscious use of off-the-shelf tools like TextBlob or Pattern, their quality for sentiment analysis of clinical narratives still has to be assessed. Information on their quality could also contribute to trust in the technology. A benchmark and a standard evaluation procedure could hold together with an annotated dataset to test and compare the quality of such tools.

18.4 Towards Understandable and Ethical Sentiment Analysis

Algorithmovigilance refers to the monitoring and evaluation of algorithms and artificial intelligence systems to ensure that their functioning is correct and ethically [58]. This involves assessing the performance and bias of the algorithm, as well as ensuring that it is being used responsibly and in accordance with relevant regulations and guidelines. Algorithmovigilance is an important aspect of the responsible development and deployment of artificial intelligence systems, particularly in fields such as healthcare, where the decisions made by algorithms can have significant consequences for individuals.

As soon as machine learning models are more frequently applied for medical sentiment analysis, methods for making these models explicable or interpretable have to be considered [211]. An overview on XAI was given in Sect. 17.2. To summarise, to make machine learning models used for medical sentiment analysis explicable or interpretable, several strategies could be followed. Simple models, such as rule-based classifiers or linear models, are often more interpretable than complex models such as deep neural networks. Many machine learning models provide feature importance or feature relevance measures, which can help identify the most important features for a given prediction. This in turn provides insights into the aspects of a text that were most influential in determining the sentiment.

There are several tools and libraries available that can help interpret the decisions made by complex machine learning models, such as LIME (Local Interpretable Model-agnostic Explanations) and SHAP (SHapley Additive exPlanations). Visualisations, such as attention maps or decision trees, can make the decisions made by a model more understandable. A human-in-the-loop approach incorporates human feedback into the model training process. For example, a human annotator reviews the model's predictions and provides feedback, which can help improve the model's accuracy and interpretability.

18.5 Demonstrating the Benefits for Patient Care

Medical sentiment analysis is not yet integrated in clinical practice, even though it is an active research fields and methods are often applied to learn more about diseases in particular from medical social media. Besides their integration into clinical decision support systems, its potentials within concrete clinical use cases has to be demonstrated. Some work has been done in the context of analysing clinical notes or other clinical narratives for predicting re-admission risk or outcomes [87]. However, this research is still in its beginnings and more convincing results have to be provided.

Several areas exist where the benefits of medical sentiment analysis for patient care can be demonstrated. Medical sentiment analysis can help identify areas of care that are particularly important to patients when used for analysing patient feedback. Accordingly, opportunities for improvement in care could be identified. This can ultimately lead to increased patient satisfaction.

Furthermore, medical sentiment analysis can be used to identify negative sentiment of patients or dissatisfaction with care, which may indicate potential safety concerns. Also patterns in patient communication that may indicate a need for additional support or follow-up could be studied, similar as it is done with medical social media data. By proactively addressing detected issues, healthcare providers can improve patient safety and communication with patients.

We recognised many use cases of medical sentiment analysis. Studies are missing that clearly show the benefits from an outcome perspective (e.g. less re-admissions of patients since critical patients were specifically monitored). To realise this, sentiment analysis-based predictions would have to be integrated into clinical decision making and randomised controlled trials have to be conducted. Beyond, the ethical concerns and unintended consequences need to be carefully addressed.

18.6 Concluding Remarks

In conclusion, the field of medical sentiment analysis is evolving and presents many opportunities for research and development. As we continue to push the boundaries of what is possible with natural language processing and machine learning, it is important to remember the quote of nobel prize winner Roger Penrose: "Don't let the lack of a perfect tool be the obstacle to reaching your goal." While there may be limitations and challenges in the current tools and techniques, it is important to continue pushing forward and finding new ways to overcome these obstacles in order to make use of the valuable information that is still often captured in medical texts. I look forward to seeing the advancements and breakthroughs that will come from the ongoing research in this area.

Glossary

Artificial neural network An artificial neural network is a type of machine learning model inspired by the structure and function of the brain. It consists of a large number of interconnected processing nodes, called artificial neurons, which work together to process and analyse complex data inputs. Each layer of interconnected neurons realises a specific task. The input layer receives the raw data, and the output layer produces the final result. One or more hidden layers between the input and output layers perform intermediate processing on the data. The connections between the neurons are weighted, and the weights are adjusted during the training process in order to improve the accuracy of the model. During training, a big dataset is fed into the neural network, and the weights are adjusted based on the difference between the predicted and actual results.

Clinical narrative A clinical narrative is a written document on a patient's medical history, treatment, and progress. It documents and communicates information about a patient's care, and may include details such as patient's symptoms, diagnosis, treatments, and clinical outcomes. Several types of clinical narratives exist reflecting the patient journey, e.g. radiology reports, nursing notes or discharge summaries.

Clinical outcome A clinical outcome is a measure of the effectiveness of a medical treatment or intervention in achieving a desired result. It can be both objective (e.g., a reduction in blood pressure or cholesterol levels) and subjective (e.g., a patient's self-reported improvement in quality of life). In clinical research, clinical outcomes are typically the primary or secondary endpoints of a study. Clinical outcomes are often used to evaluate the safety and effectiveness of a new medical treatment or intervention, and they are typically measured using standardised tools and methods.

Cognitive behaviour therapy Cognitive behaviour therapy (CBT) is a type of psychotherapy that aims to help individuals change negative patterns of thought and behaviour that may be contributing to their mental health problems. CBT is based on the idea that our thoughts, emotions, and behaviours are all

K. Denecke, *Sentiment Analysis in the Medical Domain*,
https://doi.org/10.1007/978-3-031-30187-2

interconnected, and that negative patterns in one area can contribute to difficulties in the others. CBT is often used to treat a wide range of mental health issues, including depression, anxiety, and substance abuse.

Conversational agent A conversational agent, also known as a chatbot or virtual assistant, is a computer program designed to communicate with humans in a natural language, either through text or voice interactions. They are used in a variety of applications, including customer service, entertainment or healthcare. They are accessible through websites, messaging platforms, and mobile apps. Conversational agents use natural language processing technology to understand and respond to user inputs. They can realise a wide range of tasks, including answering questions, providing information, or making recommendations.

Coreference resolution Coreference resolution is the task of identifying and linking words or phrases in a text that refer to the same entity.

Deep learning Deep learning is a subfield of machine learning that is inspired by the structure and function of the brain, specifically the neural networks that make up the brain. It involves the use of artificial neural networks used to process and analyse large amounts of data. Deep learning algorithms are designed to self-learn from large, complex datasets, i.e. to improve their performance over time without explicit programming.

Emotion recognition Emotion recognition, as opposed to sentiment analysis, identifies the emotion a person is experiencing or expressing. This emotion is typically categorised as one of several categories, such as joyful, good, angry, sorrowful, fearful, evil, and surprised [186].

Digital exposome The term "digital exposome" describes the collection of digital data and information that users create as they engage with digital platforms and devices. This includes information from social media, internet searches, shopping behaviours, and other types of digital activity.

Digital health intervention A digital health intervention is a type of health intervention that uses digital technologies, such as software, mobile apps, and wearable devices, to improve health outcomes. An example is a mobile app that tracks physical activity, nutrition, and other health behaviours. Digital health interventions can offer a number of benefits, including increased adherence, accessibility, and cost-effectiveness.

Electronic health record An electronic health record (EHR) is an electronic version of a patient's medical history, including relevant healthcare-related information such as medical diagnoses, treatments or prescribed medications. EHRs are designed to improve the efficiency and accuracy of healthcare delivery by providing a comprehensive and up-to-date record of a patient's health history.

ICD-10 The International Classification of Diseases, Tenth Revision (ICD-10) is a standardised system for classifying diseases and other health-related conditions. It is developed and maintained by the World Health Organisation (WHO) and is used to code and classify a wide range of diseases, disorders, injuries, and other health-related conditions. It consists of a set of codes and corresponding descriptions that are used to describe and classify health conditions.

Intensity classification Intensity classification is the process of assigning a level of intensity to a particular sentiment.

Irony Irony is a figure of speech used to saying or writing one thing but meaning something else, often in a humorous or sarcastic way. Irony is often used to add humour or to convey a sense of absurdity or incongruity.

Level of analysis Sentiment can be studied at different levels: Document-, sentence- or aspect-level. Depending on the level, the complexity of the analysis task differs.

Machine learning Machine learning is a subfield of artificial intelligence (AI) that involves the development of algorithms and models that can learn and improve their performance over time. Machine learning algorithms are designed to analyse data, identify patterns, and make decisions or predictions based on that data. There are different types of machine learning algorithms, including supervised learning algorithms, unsupervised learning algorithms, and reinforcement learning algorithms. Supervised learning algorithms involve training a model on a labelled dataset, where the correct output is provided for each input. The model uses this training data to learn to predict the correct output for new, unseen data. Unsupervised learning algorithms do not have labelled training data and instead try to find patterns and relationships in the data on their own.

Medical sentiment Medical sentiment is an attitude, thought, or judgement promoted by an observation with respect to the health of some individual.

Medical sentiment analysis Medical sentiment analysis is the process of using natural language processing and AI to identify and interpret the sentiment or emotion expressed in text. Medical sentiment analysis is a growing area of research and has the potential to provide valuable insights into the attitudes and experiences of patients and healthcare providers.

MetaMap MetaMap is a natural language processing tool developed by the National Library of Medicine that is used to extract biomedical concepts from text. It aims at identifying and categorising medical terms and concepts in unstructured text. MetaMap is available as a standalone tool and as part of the NLM's Unified Medical Language System (UMLS), a comprehensive resource for biomedical terminology and concepts.

mHealth mHealth or mobile health is the use of mobile technologies, such as smartphones, tablets, and wearable devices, to deliver healthcare services, information, and support. mHealth can be used to promote healthy behaviours, prevent or manage chronic conditions, and deliver clinical care.

Natural language processing (NLP) Natural language processing (NLP) is a field of artificial intelligence and computational linguistics that focuses on enabling computers to process, understand, and generate human-like language. NLP technologies are used in a wide range of applications, including language translation, text summarisation, chatbots, and voice recognition. At its core, NLP involves the development of algorithms and models that can analyse, interpret, and generate human language data. To achieve these tasks, NLP algorithms often rely on techniques from machine learning and computational linguistics, such as parsing, part-of-speech tagging, and named entity recognition. These techniques help the algorithms understand the structure and meaning of language data, and enable them to perform tasks such as language translation and text classification.

Negation A negation is a word or phrase that reverses or denies the meaning of a word or phrase.

Part-of-speech (POS) A POS (also word class or lexical category) is a linguistic category of words that have similar grammatical properties. Most languages have a set of core POS, which form sentences. These typically include nouns, verbs, adjectives, adverbs, pronouns, and prepositions.

Part-of-speech tagging Part of speech tagging is the process of annotating words with their word class, i.e. their parts-of-speech.

Pharmacovigilance Pharmacovigilance comprises activities related to detecting, assessing, understanding, and preventing adverse effects or other problems related to medications. Its objective is to ensure the safe and effective use of drugs. Pharmacovigilance activities include:

- Identifying and assessing potential risks associated with drugs,
- Monitoring the safety of drugs after they have been approved for use,
- Providing information to healthcare professionals, patients, and the public about the potential risks and benefits of drugs,
- Developing and implementing strategies to minimise the risk of harm from drugs.

Polarity Polarity refers to the sentiment orientation which can be positive, negative or neutral.

Risk factor A risk factor is a characteristic or condition that increases the likelihood of a person developing a particular health condition or disease. Examples are smoking or tobacco use, overweight or obesity. Risk factors can be modifiable, meaning that they can be changed or modified through lifestyle changes or medical interventions, or non-modifiable, meaning that they cannot be changed.

Sarcasm Sarcasm is a form of irony that involves saying or writing something that is opposite or contradictory to what one actually means, often in a humorous or mocking way. It can be used to convey negative emotions or criticism.

Sentiment lexicon A sentiment lexicon is a list of words or phrases that are associated with a specific sentiment (e.g. positive, neutral, negative) or emotion (e.g. fear, sad) or a polarity score. They can be created manually by annotating a list of words with their associated sentiment, or they can be generated automatically from large datasets of annotated text.

SNOMED CT SNOMED CT (Systematised Nomenclature of Medicine—Clinical Terms) is a comprehensive standardised vocabulary for healthcare terminology. It is used for the indexing, storage, retrieval, and interchange of clinical health data and is designed to support the electronic exchange of clinical health information. It covers a wide range of medical concepts, including diseases, disorders, procedures, substances, and other health-related terms.

Social media Social media refers to online platforms that allow people to connect with each other and share content. Some examples of social media platforms include Facebook, Twitter, Instagram, LinkedIn, and TikTok.

Subjectivity analysis Subjectivity quantifies the amount of opinionated and factual information in a text. Correspondingly, subjectivity analysis distinguishes factual from opinionated sentences or document.

Tasks of sentiment analysis Different tasks of sentiment analysis can be distinguished: Subjectivity analysis, polarity analysis, intensity classification, emotion analysis.

Unified Medical Language System (UMLS) The UMLS integrates and distributes key biomedical terminology, classification and coding standards and provides associated resources. It is curated by the National Library of Medicine.

References

1. Al-Rawi, A., Grépin, K.A., Li, X., Morgan, R., Wenham, C., Smith, J.: Investigating public discourses around gender and covid-19: a social media analysis of twitter data. J. Healthcare Inf. Res. **5**, 249–269 (2021)
2. Aladağ, A.E., Muderrisoglu, S., Akbas, N.B., Zahmacioglu, O., Bingol, H.O.: Detecting suicidal ideation on forums: proof-of-concept study. J. Med. Internet Res. **20**(6), e9840 (2018)
3. Aronson, A.R.: Metamap: Mapping text to the umls metathesaurus. Bethesda, MD: NLM, NIH, DHHS **1**, 26 (2006)
4. Ascher, J., Höglund, D., Mlika, A., Ostojic, I., Vancauwenberghe, M.: From product to customer experience: The new way to launch in pharma. McKinsey (2018). https://www.mckinsey.com/industries/pharmaceuticals-and-medical-products/our-insights/from-product-to-customer-experience-the-new-way-to-launch-in-pharma
5. Asghar, M.Z., Ahmad, S., Qasim, M., Zahra, S.R., Kundi, F.M.: Sentihealth: creating health-related sentiment lexicon using hybrid approach. SpringerPlus **5**, 1 (2016)
6. Baccianella, S., Esuli, A., Sebastiani, F.: SentiWordNet 3.0: an enhanced lexical resource for sentiment analysis and opinion mining. In: Proceedings of the Seventh International Conference on Language Resources and Evaluation (LREC'10). European Language Resources Association (ELRA), Valletta (2010)
7. Bahja, M., Lycett, M.: Identifying patient experience from online resources via sentiment analysis and topic modelling. In: Proceedings of the 3rd IEEE/ACM International Conference on Big Data Computing, Applications and Technologies, pp. 94–99 (2016). https://doi.org/10.1145/3006299.3006335
8. Balthazar, P., Harri, P., Prater, A., Safdar, N.M.: Protecting your patients' interests in the era of big data, artificial intelligence, and predictive analytics. J. Am. Coll. Radiol. **15**(3), 580–586 (2018)
9. Bansal, A., Kumar, N.: Aspect-based sentiment analysis using attribute extraction of hospital reviews. New Gener. Comput. **40**, 941–960 (2022)
10. Barbounaki, S., Gourounti, K., Sarantaki, A.: Advances of sentiment analysis applications in obstetrics/gynecology and midwifery. Mater. Socio-Med. **33**, 225–230 (2021)
11. Barkur, G., Vibha, G.B.K.: Sentiment analysis of nationwide lockdown due to covid 19 outbreak: Evidence from India. Asian J. Psychiatry **15**, 102089 (2020)
12. Bearse, P., Manejwala, O., Mohammad, A.F., Haque, I.R.I.: An initial feasibility study to identify loneliness among mental health patients from clinical notes. In: 2020 3rd International Conference on Information and Computer Technologies (ICICT), pp. 68–77 (2020). https://doi.org/10.1109/ICICT50521.2020.00019

K. Denecke, *Sentiment Analysis in the Medical Domain*,
https://doi.org/10.1007/978-3-031-30187-2

13. Beauchamp, T.L.: Methods and principles in biomedical ethics. J. Med. Ethics **29**(5), 269–274 (2003)
14. Belle, V., Papantonis, I.: Principles and practice of explainable machine learning. Front. Big Data **4**, 688969
15. Bester, J.C.: Beneficence, interests, and wellbeing in medicine: what it means to provide benefit to patients. Am. J. Bioethics **20**(3), 53–62 (2020)
16. Beykikhoshk, A., Arandjelović, O., Phung, D., Venkatesh, S., Caelli, T.: Using twitter to learn about the autism community. Soc. Netw. Anal. Min. **5**(1), 1–17 (2015)
17. Birjali, M., Kasri, M., Beni-Hssane, A.: A comprehensive survey on sentiment analysis: approaches, challenges and trends. Knowl. Based Syst. **226**, 107134 (2021). https://doi.org/10.1016/j.knosys.2021.107134. https://www.sciencedirect.com/science/article/pii/S095070512100397X
18. Blei, D.M., Ng, A.Y., Jordan, M.I.: Latent Dirichlet allocation. J. Mach. Learn. Res. **3**, 993–1022 (2003)
19. Blobel, B., Ruotsalainen, P., Brochhausen, M.: Autonomous systems and artificial intelligence-hype or prerequisite for p5 medicine? In: pHealth, pp. 3–14 (2021)
20. Bodenreider, O.: The unified medical language system (UMLS): integrating biomedical terminology. Nucleic Acids Res. **32**(suppl_1), D267–D270 (2004)
21. Boonitt, S., Skunkan, Y.: Public perception of the covid-19 pandemic on twitter: Sentiment analysis and topic modeling study. JMIR Public Health Surveill. **6**, e21978 (2020)
22. Brezulianu, A., Burlacu, A., Popa, I.V., Arif, M., Geman, O.: "not by our feeling, but by other's seeing": Sentiment analysis technique in cardiology–an exploratory review. Front. Public Health **10**, 880207 (2022)
23. Cabling, M.L., Turner, J.W., Hurtado-de Mendoza, A., Zhang, Y., Jiang, X., Drago, F., Sheppard, V.B.: Sentiment analysis of an online breast cancer support group: communicating about tamoxifen. Health Commun. **33**(9), 1158–1165 (2018)
24. Caillot, O., Aubry, M., Duros, S., Boyer, L., Van Valenberg, C., Levêque, J., Lavoué, V.: Impact of the French 3rd and 4th generation pill scare in women seeking termination of pregnancy. J. Gynecol. Obstet. Human Reprod. **46**(1), 69–76 (2017)
25. Caliskan, A., Bryson, J.J., Narayanan, A.: Semantics derived automatically from language corpora contain human-like biases. Science **356**(6334), 183–186 (2017)
26. Cambria, E.: Affective computing and sentiment analysis. IEEE Intell. Syst. **31**(2), 102–107 (2016)
27. Carchiolo, V., Longheu, A., Malgeri, M.: Using twitter data and sentiment analysis to study diseases dynamics. In: International Conference on Information Technology in Bio-and Medical Informatics, pp. 16–24. Springer (2015)
28. Carrillo-de Albornoz, J., Rodríguez-Vidal, J., Plaza, L.: ediseases dataset (2018). https://doi.org/10.5281/zenodo.1479354
29. Chapman, W.W., Hilert, D., Velupillai, S., Kvist, M., Skeppstedt, M., Chapman, B.E., Conway, M., Tharp, M., Mowery, D.L., Deleger, L.: Extending the negex lexicon for multiple languages. Stud. Health Technol. Inf. **192**, 677 (2013)
30. Charlesworth, T.E., Yang, V., Mann, T.C., Kurdi, B., Banaji, M.R.: Gender stereotypes in natural language: Word embeddings show robust consistency across child and adult language corpora of more than 65 million words. Psychol. Sci. **32**(2), 218–240 (2021)
31. Chatzitheodorou, K.: Improving translation memory fuzzy matching by paraphrasing. In: Proceedings of the Workshop Natural Language Processing for Translation Memories, pp. 24–30. Association for Computational Linguistics, Hissar (2015). https://aclanthology.org/W15-5204
32. Chen, Q., Sokolova, M.: Word2vec and doc2vec in unsupervised sentiment analysis of clinical discharge summaries. CoRR abs/1805.00352 (2018). http://arxiv.org/abs/1805.00352
33. Choi, S., Choi, J.: Snumedinfo at TREC CDS track 2014: Medical case-based retrieval task. In: TREC (2014)
34. Chopan, M., Sayadi, L., Clark, E.M., Maguire, K.: Plastic surgery and social media: examining perceptions. Plastic Reconstr. Surg. **143**(4), 1259–1265 (2019)

35. Cirillo, D., Catuara-Solarz, S., Morey, C., Guney, E., Subirats, L., Mellino, S., Gigante, A., Valencia, A., Rementeria, M.J., Chadha, A.S., et al.: Sex and gender differences and biases in artificial intelligence for biomedicine and healthcare. NPJ Digital Med. **3**(1), 1–11 (2020)
36. Clark, K., Khandelwal, U., Levy, O., Manning, C.D.: What does bert look at? An analysis of bert's attention. Preprint. arXiv:1906.04341 (2019)
37. Colón-Ruiz, C., Segura-Bedmar, I.: Comparing deep learning architectures for sentiment analysis on drug reviews. J. Biomed. Inf. **110**, 103539 (2020)
38. Craig, W., Boniel-Nissim, M., King, N., Walsh, S.D., Boer, M., Donnelly, P.D., Harel-Fisch, Y., Malinowska-Cieślik, M., de Matos, M.G., Cosma, A., et al.: Social media use and cyberbullying: a cross-national analysis of young people in 42 countries. J. Adolesc. Health **66**(6), S100–S108 (2020)
39. Crocamo, C., Viviani, M., Famiglini, L., Bartoli, F., Pasi, G., Carrà, G.: Surveilling covid-19 emotional contagion on twitter by sentiment analysis. Eur. Psychiatry **64**(1), e17 (2021). https://doi.org/10.1192/j.eurpsy.2021.3
40. Crossley, S.A., Kyle, K., McNamara, D.S.: Sentiment analysis and social cognition engine (seance): an automatic tool for sentiment, social cognition, and social-order analysis. Behav. Res. Methods **49**(3), 803–821 (2017)
41. Dang, T.T., Ho, T.B.: Mixture of language models utilization in score-based sentiment classification on clinical narratives. In: International Conference on Industrial, Engineering and Other Applications of Applied Intelligent Systems, pp. 255–268. Springer (2016)
42. de Albornoz, J.C., Vidal, J.R., Plaza, L.: Feature engineering for sentiment analysis in e-health forums. PLOS One **13**(11), 1–25 (2018)
43. de Las Heras-Pedrosa, C., Sánchez-Núñez, P., Peláez, J.I.: Sentiment analysis and emotion understanding during the covid-19 pandemic in Spain and its impact on digital ecosystems. Int. J. Environ. Res. Public Health **17**(15), 5542 (2020)
44. De Smedt, T., Daelemans, W.: Pattern for python. J. Mach. Learn. Res. **13**(66), 2063–2067 (2012)
45. del Arco, F.M.P., Valdivia, M.T.M., Zafra, S.M.J., González, M.D.M., Cámara, E.M.: Copos: corpus of patient opinions in Spanish. Application of sentiment analysis techniques. Procesamiento Lenguaje Nat. **57**, 83–90 (2016)
46. Del Canale, S., Louis, D.Z., Maio, V., Wang, X., Rossi, G., Hojat, M., Gonnella, J.S.: The relationship between physician empathy and disease complications: an empirical study of primary care physicians and their diabetic patients in Parma, Italy. Acad. Med. **87**(9), 1243–1249 (2012)
47. Denecke, K.: Using sentiwordnet for multilingual sentiment analysis. In: 2008 IEEE 24th International Conference on Data Engineering Workshop, pp. 507–512 (2008). https://doi.org/10.1109/ICDEW.2008.4498370
48. Denecke, K.: Health Web Science: Social Media Data for Healthcare. Springer (2015)
49. Denecke, K., Deng, Y.: Sentiment analysis in medical settings: new opportunities and challenges. Artif. Intell. Med. **64**(1), 17–27 (2015)
50. Denecke, K., Nejdl, W.: How valuable is medical social media data? Content analysis of the medical web. Inf. Sci. **179**(12), 1870–1880 (2009)
51. Denecke, K., May, R., Deng, Y.: Towards emotion-sensitive conversational user interfaces in healthcare applications. Stud. Health Technol. Inf. **264**, 1164–1168 (2019)
52. Denecke, K., Vaaheesan, S., Arulnathan, A.: A mental health chatbot for regulating emotions (sermo)-concept and usability test. IEEE Trans. Emerg. Top. Comput. **9**, 1170 (2020)
53. Deng, Y., Declerck, T., Lendvai, P., Denecke, K.: The generation of a corpus for clinical sentiment analysis. In: Sack, H., Rizzo, G., Steinmetz, N., Mladenić, D., Auer, S., Lange, C. (eds.) The Semantic Web, pp. 311–324. Springer International Publishing, Cham (2016)
54. Devaram, S.: Empathic chatbot: emotional intelligence for mental health well-being. ArXiv abs/2012.09130 (2020)
55. Devlin, J., Chang, M.W., Lee, K., Toutanova, K.: BERT: Pre-training of deep bidirectional transformers for language understanding. In: Proceedings of the 2019 Conference of the North American Chapter of the Association for Computational Linguistics: Human

Language Technologies, Volume 1 (Long and Short Papers), pp. 4171–4186. Association for Computational Linguistics, Minneapolis, Minnesota (2019). https://doi.org/10.18653/v1/N19-1423. https://aclanthology.org/N19-1423
56. Dodds, P.S., Harris, K.D., Kloumann, I.M., Bliss, C.A., Danforth, C.M.: Temporal patterns of happiness and information in a global social network: Hedonometrics and twitter. PloS One **6**(12), e26752 (2011)
57. ElMessiry, A., Zhang, Z., Cooper, W.O., Catron, T.F., Karrass, J., Singh, M.P.: Leveraging sentiment analysis for classifying patient complaints. In: Proceedings of the 8th ACM International Conference on Bioinformatics, Computational Biology, and Health Informatics, pp. 44–51 (2017). https://doi.org/10.1145/3107411.3107421
58. Embi, P.J.: Algorithmovigilance-advancing methods to analyze and monitor artificial intelligence-driven health care for effectiveness and equity. JAMA Netw. Open **4**(4), e214622–e214622 (2021)
59. Fiok, K., Farahani, F.V., Karwowski, W., Ahram, T.: Explainable artificial intelligence for education and training. J. Defense Model. Simul. **19**(2), 133–144 (2022)
60. Fischer, I., Steiger, H.J.: Toward automatic evaluation of medical abstracts: the current value of sentiment analysis and machine learning for classification of the importance of pubmed abstracts of randomized trials for stroke. J. Stroke Cerebrovasc. Diseases Off. J. Natl. Stroke Assoc. **29**(9), 105042 (2020)
61. Fitzpatrick, K.K., Darcy, A., Vierhile, M.: Delivering cognitive behavior therapy to young adults with symptoms of depression and anxiety using a fully automated conversational agent (Woebot): a randomized controlled trial. JMIR Mental Health **4**(2), e19 (2017)
62. Floridi, L., Cowls, J., Beltrametti, M., Chatila, R., Chazerand, P., Dignum, V., Luetge, C., Madelin, R., Pagallo, U., Rossi, F., et al.: An ethical framework for a good ai society: opportunities, risks, principles, and recommendations. In: Ethics, Governance, and Policies in Artificial Intelligence, pp. 19–39. Springer (2021)
63. Foufi, V., Timakum, T., Gaudet-Blavignac, C., Lovis, C., Song, M., et al.: Mining of textual health information from reddit: analysis of chronic diseases with extracted entities and their relations. J. Med. Internet Res. **21**(6), e12876 (2019)
64. Fulmer, R., Joerin, A., Gentile, B., Lakerink, L., Rauws, M.: Using psychological artificial intelligence (Tess) to relieve symptoms of depression and anxiety: Randomized controlled trial. JMIR Mental Health **5**, e9782 (2018)
65. Funnell, E., Spadaro, B., Martin-Key, N.A., Metcalfe, T., Bahn, S.: mhealth solutions for mental health screening and diagnosis: a review of app user perspectives using sentiment and thematic analysis. Front. Psychiatry **13**, 857304 (2022)
66. Gabarron, E., Dorronzoro, E., Rivera-Romero, O., Wynn, R.: Diabetes on twitter: a sentiment analysis. J. Diabetes Sci. Technol. **13**(3), 439–444 (2019)
67. Gabarron, E., Dechsling, A., Skafle, I., Nordahl-Hansen, A., et al.: Discussions of Asperger syndrome on social media: content and sentiment analysis on twitter. JMIR Formative Res. **6**(3), e32752 (2022)
68. Garcia-Moya, L., Anaya-Sánchez, H., Berlanga-Llavori, R.: Retrieving product features and opinions from customer reviews. IEEE Intell. Syst. **28**(3), 19–27 (2013)
69. Ghassemi, M.M., Mark, R.G., Nemati, S.: A visualization of evolving clinical sentiment using vector representations of clinical notes. In: 2015 Computing in Cardiology Conference (CinC), pp. 629–632 (2015). https://doi.org/10.1109/CIC.2015.7410989
70. Ghassemi, M.M., Al-Hanai, T., Raffa, J.D., Mark, R.G., Nemati, S., Chokshi, F.H.: How is the doctor feeling? ICU provider sentiment is associated with diagnostic imaging utilization. In: 2018 40th Annual International Conference of the IEEE Engineering in Medicine and Biology Society (EMBC), pp. 4058–4064 (2018). https://doi.org/10.1109/EMBC.2018.8513325
71. Gillon, R.: Medical ethics: four principles plus attention to scope. Bmj **309**(6948), 184 (1994)
72. Go, A., Bhayani, R., Huang, L.: Twitter sentiment classification using distant supervision. CS224N project report, Stanford **1**(12), 2009 (2009)

73. Goeuriot, L., Na, J.C., Min Kyaing, W.Y., Khoo, C., Chang, Y.K., Theng, Y.L., Kim, J.J.: Sentiment lexicons for health-related opinion mining. In: Proceedings of the 2nd ACM SIGHIT International Health Informatics Symposium, pp. 219–226 (2012)
74. Gräßer, F., Beckert, S., Küster, D., Abraham, S., Malberg, H., Schmitt, J., Zaunseder, S.: Neighborhood-based collaborative filtering for therapy decision support. In: HealthRecSys@ RecSys, pp. 22–26 (2017)
75. Gräßer, F., Kallumadi, S., Malberg, H., Zaunseder, S.: Aspect-based sentiment analysis of drug reviews applying cross-domain and cross-data learning. In: Proceedings of the 2018 International Conference on Digital Health, pp. 121–125 (2018). https://doi.org/10.1145/3194658.3194677
76. Greaves, F., Ramirez-Cano, D., Millett, C., Darzi, A., Donaldson, L., et al.: Use of sentiment analysis for capturing patient experience from free-text comments posted online. J. Med. Internet Res. **15**(11), e2721 (2013)
77. Grisstte, H., Nfaoui, E.: Daily life patients sentiment analysis model based on well-encoded embedding vocabulary for related-medication text. In: Proceedings of the 2019 IEEE/ACM International Conference on Advances in Social Networks Analysis and Mining, pp. 921–928 (2019). https://doi.org/10.1145/3341161.3343854
78. Grissette, H., Nfaoui, E.H., Bahir, A.: Sentiment analysis tool for pharmaceutical industry & healthcare. Trans. Mach. Learn. Artif. Intell. **5**(4) (2017). https://doi.org/10.14738/tmlai.54.3339
79. Guarita, B., Belackova, V., Van Der Gouwe, D., Blankers, M., Pazitny, M., Griffiths, P.: Monitoring drug trends in the digital environment–new methods, challenges and the opportunities provided by automated approaches. Int. J. Drug Policy **94**, 103210 (2021)
80. Guntuku, S.C., Buffone, A., Jaidka, K., Eichstaedt, J.C., Ungar, L.H.: Understanding and measuring psychological stress using social media. In: ICWSM (2019)
81. Gupta, R., Vishwanath, A., Yang, Y.: Global reactions to covid-19 on twitter: a labelled dataset with latent topic, sentiment and emotion attributes. arXiv:2007.06954v6 (2021)
82. Hansson, M.G.: Ethics and biobanks. Br. J. Cancer **100**(1), 8–12 (2009)
83. Hase, P., Bansal, M.: Evaluating explainable AI: Which algorithmic explanations help users predict model behavior? Preprint. arXiv:2005.01831 (2020)
84. Hemalatha, R., Monicka, M.B.: Sentiment analysis on myocardial infarction using tweets data. Int. J. Comput. Sci. Technol. **9**(4), 61–65 (2018)
85. Hickson, G.B., Caruso-Hayden, A.C., Pichert, J.W.: The pars® program: How unsolicited patient comments can be used to promote a safer healthcare environment, address unprofessional conduct and reduce unnecessary malpractice risk. In: Annual Meeting of the American Health Lawyers Association. Seattle (2010)
86. Holderness, E., Cawkwell, P., Bolton, K., Meteer, M., Pustejovsky, J., Hall, M.H.: S180. defining clinical sentiment in psychosis patient health records. Biological Psychiatry **85**(10), S367 (2019)
87. Holderness, E., Cawkwell, P., Bolton, K., Pustejovsky, J., Hall, M.H.: Distinguishing clinical sentiment: The importance of domain adaptation in psychiatric patient health records. In: Proceedings of the 2nd Clinical Natural Language Processing Workshop, pp. 117–123. Association for Computational Linguistics, Minneapolis, Minnesota (2019). https://doi.org/10.18653/v1/W19-1915. https://aclanthology.org/W19-1915
88. Holzinger, A., Saranti, A., Molnar, C., Biecek, P., Samek, W.: Explainable AI methods-a brief overview. In: International Workshop on Extending Explainable AI Beyond Deep Models and Classifiers, pp. 13–38. Springer (2022)
89. Hsu, D., Moh, M., Moh, T.S.: Mining frequency of drug side effects over a large twitter dataset using apache spark. In: Proceedings of the 2017 IEEE/ACM International Conference on Advances in Social Networks Analysis and Mining 2017, pp. 915–924 (2017). https://doi.org/10.1145/3110025.3110110
90. Htet, H., Myint, Y.Y.: Social media (Twitter) data analysis using maximum entropy classifier on big data processing framework (case study: Analysis of health condition, education status, states of business). Ph.D. thesis, MERAL Portal (2018)

91. Hu, M., Liu, B.: Mining and summarizing customer reviews. In: Proceedings of the tenth ACM SIGKDD international conference on Knowledge discovery and data mining, pp. 168–177 (2004)
92. Hurst, S.: Eigentümer seiner selbst. Ethische Implikationen von Autonomie im digitalen Zeitalter. In: Autonomie und Digitalisierung. Ein neues Kapitel für die Selbstbestimmung in der Medizin? Bericht zur Tagung vom 15. Juni 2018 des Veranstaltungszyklus "Autonomie in der Medizin". Edited by: Schweizerische Akademie der Medizinischen Wissenschaften, SAMW; Brauer, Susanne; Strub, Jean-Daniel; Büchler, Andrea; et al., vol. 13, Nr. 7, pp. 41–45. Bern: Schweizerische Akademie der Medizinischen Wissenschaften (SAMW) (2018)
93. Hussein, A., Ahmad, F.K., Kamaruddin, S.S.: Cluster analysis on covid-19 outbreak sentiments from twitter data using k-means algorithm. J. Syst. Manag. Sci. **11**(4), 167–189 (2021)
94. Hutto, C., Gilbert, E.: Vader: A parsimonious rule-based model for sentiment analysis of social media text. In: Proceedings of the International AAAI Conference on Web and Social Media, vol. 8(1), pp. 216–225 (2014)
95. Imran, A.S., Daudpota, S.M., Kastrati, Z., Batra, R.: Cross-cultural polarity and emotion detection using sentiment analysis and deep learning on covid-19 related tweets. IEEE Access **8**, 181074–181090 (2020)
96. Insel, T.R.: Digital phenotyping: a global tool for psychiatry. World Psychiatry **17**(3), 276 (2018)
97. Jiménez-Zafra, S.M., Martín-Valdivia, M.T., Molina-González, M.D., Ureña-López, L.A.: How do we talk about doctors and drugs? Sentiment analysis in forums expressing opinions for medical domain. Artif. Intell. Med. **93**, 50–57 (2019)
98. Jindal, N., Liu, B.: Opinion spam and analysis. In: Proceedings of the 2008 International Conference on Web Search and Data Mining, pp. 219–230 (2008)
99. Johnson, A.E.W., Pollard, T.J., Shen, L., wei H. Lehman, L., Feng, M., Ghassemi, M.M., Moody, B., Szolovits, P., Celi, L.A., Mark, R.G.: MIMIC-III, a freely accessible critical care database. Sci. Data **3**, 1 (2016)
100. Johnson, A.E., Pollard, T.J., Berkowitz, S.J., Greenbaum, N.R., Lungren, M.P., Deng, C.y., Mark, R.G., Horng, S.: MIMIC-CXR, a de-identified publicly available database of chest radiographs with free-text reports. Sci. Data **6**(1), 1–8 (2019)
101. Johnson, A., Bulgarelli, L., Pollard, T., Celi, L.A., Mark, R., Horng, S.: MIMIC-IV-ED. In: PhsyioNet (2022)
102. Jung, Y., Hur, C., Jung, D., Kim, M.: Identifying key hospital service quality factors in online health communities. J. Med. Internet Res. **17**(4), e90 (2015)
103. Jurafsky, D., Martin, J.H.: Speech and Language Processing: An Introduction to Natural Language Processing, Computational Linguistics and Speech Recognition, 2nd edn., [pearson international edition] edn. Prentice Hall Series in Artificial Intelligence. Prentice Hall, Pearson Education International, Englewood Cliffs, NJ (2009)
104. Kaufman, L.M.: Data security in the world of cloud computing. IEEE Secur. Privacy **7**(4), 61–64 (2009)
105. Khan, A., Asghar, M.Z., Ahmad, H., Kundi, F.M., Ismail, S.: A rule-based sentiment classification framework for health reviews on mobile social media. J. Med. Imaging Health Inf. **7**(6), 1445–1453 (2017)
106. Knapp, A., Harst, L., Hager, S., Schmitt, J., Scheibe, M., et al.: Use of patient-reported outcome measures and patient-reported experience measures within evaluation studies of telemedicine applications: systematic review. J. Med. Internet Res. **23**(11), e30042 (2021)
107. Kumar, C.S.P., Babu, L.D.D.: Evolving dictionary based sentiment scoring framework for patient authored text. Evol. Intell. **14**(2), 657–667 (2021)
108. LaRosa, E., Danks, D.: Impacts on trust of healthcare AI. In: Proceedings of the 2018 AAAI/ACM Conference on AI, Ethics, and Society, pp. 210–215 (2018)
109. Levis, M., Westgate, C.L., Gui, J., Watts, B.V., Shiner, B.: Natural language processing of clinical mental health notes may add predictive value to existing suicide risk models. Psychol. Med. **51**(8), 1382–1391 (2021)

110. Li, Y., Su, H., Shen, X., Li, W., Cao, Z., Niu, S.: Dailydialog: a manually labelled multi-turn dialogue dataset. Preprint. arXiv:1710.03957 (2017)
111. Li, J., Zhou, Y., Jiang, X., Natarajan, K., Pakhomov, S.V., Liu, H., Xu, H.: Are synthetic clinical notes useful for real natural language processing tasks: a case study on clinical entity recognition. J. Am. Med. Inf. Assoc. **28**(10), 2193–2201 (2021)
112. Ligthart, A., Catal, C., Tekinerdogan, B.: Systematic reviews in sentiment analysis: a tertiary study. Artif. Intell. Rev. **54**(7), 4997–5053 (2021)
113. Lin, S., Su, W., Chien, P., Tsai, M., Wang, C.: Self-attentive sentimental sentence embedding for sentiment analysis. In: ICASSP 2020 - 2020 IEEE International Conference on Acoustics, Speech and Signal Processing (ICASSP), pp. 1678–1682 (2020)
114. Liu, B.: Sentiment analysis and opinion mining. Synthesis Lectures on Human Language Technologies, vol. 5(1), pp. 1–167 (2012)
115. Liu, B.: Many Facets of Sentiment Analysis, pp. 11–39. Springer International Publishing, Cham (2017)
116. Liu, X., Chen, H.: Identifying adverse drug events from patient social media: a case study for diabetes. IEEE Intell. Syst. **30**(3), 44–51 (2015)
117. Liu, S., Lee, I.: Extracting features with medical sentiment lexicon and position encoding for drug reviews. Health Inf. Sci. Syst. **7**(1), 1–10 (2019)
118. Liu, B., Hu, M., Cheng, J.: Opinion observer: analyzing and comparing opinions on the web. In: Proceedings of the 14th International Conference on World Wide Web, pp. 342–351 (2005)
119. Liu, Z., Dong, X., Guan, Y., Yang, J.: Reserved self-training: a semi-supervised sentiment classification method for Chinese microblogs. In: Proceedings of the Sixth International Joint Conference on Natural Language Processing, pp. 455–462 (2013)
120. Liu, J., Zhang, W., Jiang, X., Zhou, Y.: Data mining of the reviews from online private doctors. Telemedicine e-Health **26**(9), 1157–1166 (2020)
121. Liu, T., Meyerhoff, J., Eichstaedt, J.C., Karr, C.J., Kaiser, S.M., Kording, K.P., Mohr, D.C., Kulkarni, P.V.: The relationship between text message sentiment and self-reported depression. J. Affective Disord. **302**, 7 (2021)
122. Lowres, N., Duckworth, A., Redfern, J., Thiagalingam, A., Chow, C.K.: Use of a machine learning program to correctly triage incoming text messaging replies from a cardiovascular text-based secondary prevention program: feasibility study. JMIR mHealth uHealth **8**, e19200 (2020)
123. Madasu, A., Elango, S.: Efficient feature selection techniques for sentiment analysis. Multimed. Tools Appl. **79**, 6313–6335 (2020)
124. Mammen, J.R., Elson, M.J., Java, J.J., Beck, C.A., Beran, D.B., Biglan, K.M., Boyd, C.M., Schmidt, P.N., Simone, R., Willis, A.W., et al.: Patient and physician perceptions of virtual visits for Parkinson's disease: a qualitative study. Telemed. e-Health **24**(4), 255–267 (2018)
125. Marelli, L., Lievevrouw, E., Van Hoyweghen, I.: Fit for purpose? The GDPR and the governance of European digital health. Policy Stud. **41**(5), 447–467 (2020)
126. Matošević, G., Bevanda, V.: Sentiment analysis of tweets about covid-19 disease during pandemic. In: 2020 43rd International Convention on Information, Communication and Electronic Technology (MIPRO), pp. 1290–1295 (2020). https://doi.org/10.23919/MIPRO48935.2020.9245176
127. McCoy, T.H., Castro, V.M., Cagan, A., Roberson, A.M., Kohane, I.S., Perlis, R.H.: Sentiment measured in hospital discharge notes is associated with readmission and mortality risk: an electronic health record study. PLoS One **10**, e0136341 (2015)
128. McDonnell, M., Owen, J.E., Bantum, E.O., et al.: Identification of emotional expression with cancer survivors: validation of linguistic inquiry and word count. JMIR Formative Res. **4**(10), e18246 (2020)
129. Mehrabi, S., Krishnan, A., Sohn, S., Roch, A.M., Schmidt, H., Kesterson, J., Beesley, C., Dexter, P., Schmidt, C.M., Liu, H., et al.: DEEPEN: a negation detection system for clinical text incorporating dependency relation into NegEx. J. Biomed. Inf. **54**, 213–219 (2015)
130. Mellado, E.Á., Holderness, E., Miller, N., Dhang, F., Cawkwell, P.B., Bolton, K., Pustejovsky, J., Hall, M.H.: Assessing the efficacy of clinical sentiment analysis and topic extraction in psychiatric readmission risk prediction. ArXiv abs/1910.04006 (2019)

131. Mike, T., Kevan, B., Georgios, P., Di, C.: Sentiment in short strength detection informal text. JASIST **61**(12), 2544–2558 (2010)
132. Mikolov, T., Sutskever, I., Chen, K., Corrado, G., Dean, J.: Distributed representations of words and phrases and their compositionality. In: Proceedings of the 26th International Conference on Neural Information Processing Systems - Volume 2, NIPS'13, pp. 3111–3119. Curran Associates Inc., Red Hook, NY (2013)
133. Mishra, A., Malviya, A., Aggarwal, S.: Towards automatic pharmacovigilance: analysing patient reviews and sentiment on oncological drugs. In: 2015 IEEE International Conference on Data Mining Workshop (ICDMW), pp. 1402–1409 (2015). https://doi.org/10.1109/ICDMW.2015.230
134. Mizan Khairul Anwar, M.K., Yusoff, M., Kassim, M.: Decision tree and naïve bayes for sentiment analysis in smoking perception. In: 2022 IEEE 12th Symposium on Computer Applications & Industrial Electronics (ISCAIE), pp. 294–299 (2022). https://doi.org/10.1109/ISCAIE54458.2022.9794558
135. Mohammad, S.M.: Practical and ethical considerations in the effective use of emotion and sentiment lexicons. Preprint. arXiv:2011.03492 (2020)
136. Mohammad, S.M.: Ethics sheet for automatic emotion recognition and sentiment analysis. Comput. Linguist. **48**(2), 239–278 (2022)
137. Mohammad, S.M., Bravo-Marquez, F.: Wassa-2017 shared task on emotion intensity. Preprint. arXiv:1708.03700 (2017)
138. Mohammad, S.M., Turney, P.D.: Crowdsourcing a word–emotion association lexicon. Comput. Intell. **29**(3), 436–465 (2013)
139. Mohammad, S., Dunne, C., Dorr, B.: Generating high-coverage semantic orientation lexicons from overtly marked words and a thesaurus. In: Proceedings of the 2009 Conference on Empirical Methods in Natural Language Processing, pp. 599–608 (2009)
140. Mohan, M., Abhinav, A.K., Ashok, A., Akhil, A.V., Achinth, P.R.: Depression detection using facial expression and sentiment analysis. In: 2021 Asian Conference on Innovation in Technology (ASIANCON), pp. 1–6 (2021). https://doi.org/10.1109/ASIANCON51346.2021.9544819
141. Mondal, A., Das, D.: Ensemble approach for identifying medical concepts with special attention to lexical scope. Sādhanā **46**(2), 1–12 (2021)
142. Mondal, A., Das, D., Cambria, E., Bandyopadhyay, S.: WME: sense, polarity and affinity based concept resource for medical events. In: Proceedings of the 8th Global WordNet Conference (GWC), pp. 243–248. Global Wordnet Association, Bucharest (2016). https://aclanthology.org/2016.gwc-1.35
143. Mondal, A., Cambria, E., Das, D., Hussain, A., Bandyopadhyay, S.: Relation extraction of medical concepts using categorization and sentiment analysis. Cogn. Comput. **10**(4), 670–685 (2018)
144. Mondal, A., Das, D., Cambria, E., Bandyopadhyay, S.: WME 3.0: an enhanced and validated lexicon of medical concepts. In: Proceedings of the 9th Global Wordnet Conference, pp. 10–16. Global Wordnet Association, Nanyang Technological University (NTU), Singapore (2018). https://aclanthology.org/2018.gwc-1.2
145. Müller, M., Salathé, M., Kummervold, P.E.: Covid-twitter-bert: a natural language processing model to analyse covid-19 content on twitter. Preprint. arXiv:2005.07503 (2020)
146. Mummalaneni, V., Gruss, R., Goldberg, D.M., Ehsani, J.P., Abrahams, A.S.: Social media analytics for quality surveillance and safety hazard detection in baby cribs. Safety Sci. **104**, 260–268 (2018)
147. Munezero, M.D., Montero, C.S., Sutinen, E., Pajunen, J.: Are they different? Affect, feeling, emotion, sentiment, and opinion detection in text. IEEE Trans. Affective Comput. **5**(2), 101–111 (2014)
148. Nandwani, P., Verma, R.: A review on sentiment analysis and emotion detection from text. Soc. Netw. Anal. Min. **11**(1), 1–19 (2021)
149. Nazir, A., Rao, Y., Wu, L., Sun, L.: Issues and challenges of aspect-based sentiment analysis: a comprehensive survey. IEEE Trans. Affect. Comput. **13**(2), 845–863 (2022)

150. Nielsen, F.Å.: A new anew: evaluation of a word list for sentiment analysis in microblogs. Preprint. arXiv:1103.2903 (2011)
151. Niu, Y., Zhu, X., Li, J., Hirst, G.: Analysis of polarity information in medical text. In: AMIA annual symposium proceedings, vol. 2005, p. 570. American Medical Informatics Association (2005)
152. O'dea, B., Larsen, M.E., Batterham, P.J., Calear, A.L., Christensen, H.: A linguistic analysis of suicide-related twitter posts. Crisis **38**(5), 319 (2017)
153. O'Neill, O.: Accountability, trust and informed consent in medical practice and research. Clin. Med. **4**(3), 269 (2004)
154. of Michigan, U.: Kaggle. UMICH SI650 - sentiment classification (2018). https://www.kaggle.com/c/si650winter11
155. Onyimadu, O., Nakata, K., Wilson, T., Macken, D., Liu, K.: Towards sentiment analysis on parliamentary debates in Hansard. In: Joint International Semantic Technology Conference, pp. 48–50. Springer (2013)
156. Pandesenda, A.I., Yana, R.R., Sukma, E.A., Yahya, A.N., Widharto, P., Hidayanto, A.N.: Sentiment analysis of service quality of online healthcare platform using fast large-margin. In: 2020 International Conference on Informatics, Multimedia, Cyber and Information System (ICIMCIS), pp. 121–125 (2020)
157. Peng, Y., Moh, M., Moh, T.S.: Efficient adverse drug event extraction using twitter sentiment analysis. In: Proceedings of the 2016 IEEE/ACM International Conference on Advances in Social Networks Analysis and Mining, pp. 1011–1018 (2016)
158. Pérez, K.C., Sánchez-Cervantes, J.L., del Pilar Salas-Zárate, M., Hernández, L.Á.R., Rodríguez-Mazahua, L.: A sentiment analysis approach for drug reviews in Spanish. Res. Comput. Sci. **149**(5), 43–51 (2020)
159. Pestian, J.P., Matykiewicz, P., Linn-Gust, M., South, B., Uzuner, O., Wiebe, J., Cohen, K.B., Hurdle, J., Brew, C.: Sentiment analysis of suicide notes: a shared task. Biomed. Inf. Insights **5**, BII–S9042 (2012)
160. Peters, M.E., Neumann, M., Iyyer, M., Gardner, M., Clark, C., Lee, K., Zettlemoyer, L.: Deep contextualized word representations. In: Proceedings of the 2018 Conference of the North American Chapter of the Association for Computational Linguistics: Human Language Technologies, Volume 1 (Long Papers), pp. 2227–2237. Association for Computational Linguistics, New Orleans, Louisiana (2018). https://doi.org/10.18653/v1/N18-1202. https://aclanthology.org/N18-1202
161. Polisena, J., Andellini, M., Salerno, P., Borsci, S., Pecchia, L., Iadanza, E.: Case studies on the use of sentiment analysis to assess the effectiveness and safety of health technologies: a scoping review. IEEE Access **9**, 66043 (2021)
162. Raghupathi, V., Ren, J., Raghupathi, W.: Studying public perception about vaccination: a sentiment analysis of tweets. Int. J. Environ. Res. Public Health **17**(10), 3464 (2020)
163. Remus, R., Quasthoff, U., Heyer, G.: Sentiws - a publicly available German-language resource for sentiment analysis. In: Proceedings of the Seventh conference on International Language Resources and Evaluation (LREC'10) (2010)
164. Ribeiro, M.T., Singh, S., Guestrin, C.: "why should i trust you?" Explaining the predictions of any classifier. In: Proceedings of the 22nd ACM SIGKDD International Conference on Knowledge Discovery and Data Mining, pp. 1135–1144 (2016)
165. Rinker, T.W.: sentimentr: Calculate text polarity sentiment. University at Buffalo/SUNY, Buffalo, New York. version 0.5, **3** (2016)
166. Rodrigues, R.G., das Dores, R.M., Camilo-Junior, C.G., Couto, T.: Sentihealth-cancer: a sentiment analysis tool to help detecting mood of patients in online social networks. Int. J. Med. Inf. **85**(1), 80–95 (2016)
167. Sabra, S., Malik, K.M., Alobaidi, M.: Prediction of venous thromboembolism using semantic and sentiment analyses of clinical narratives. Comput. Biol. Med. **94**, 1–10 (2018)
168. Samek, W., Wiegand, T., Müller, K.R.: Explainable artificial intelligence: understanding, visualizing and interpreting deep learning models. Preprint. arXiv:1708.08296 (2017)

169. Samuel, J., Ali, G., Rahman, M., Esawi, E., Samuel, Y., et al.: COVID-19 public sentiment insights and machine learning for tweets classification. SSRN Electron. J. 1–21 (2020)
170. Sanglerdsinlapachai, N., Plangprasopchok, A., Ho, T.B., Nantajeewarawat, E.: Improving sentiment analysis on clinical narratives by exploiting UMLS semantic types. Artif. Intell. Med. **113**, 102033 (2021)
171. Schmidhuber, J.: Deep learning in neural networks: an overview. Neural Netw. **61**, 85–117 (2015)
172. Seitz, L., Bekmeier-Feuerhahn, S.: Empathic healthcare chatbots: comparing the effects of emotional expression and caring behavior. In: ICIS (2021)
173. Shah, A.M., Yan, X., Shah, S.A.A., Shah, S.J., Mamirkulova, G.: Exploring the impact of online information signals in leveraging the economic returns of physicians. J. Biomed. Inf. **98**, 103272 (2019)
174. Sharma, M., Singh, G., Singh, R.: An advanced conceptual diagnostic healthcare framework for diabetes and cardiovascular disorders. EAI Endorsed Trans. Scalable Inf. Syst. **5**, e5 (2018)
175. Skorburg, J.A., Friesen, P.: Ethical issues in text mining for mental health. In: Dehghani, M., Boyd, R. (eds.) The Atlas of Language Analysis in Psychology. Guilford Press, New York (forthcoming). Preprint available at: https://philarchive.org/archive/AUGEII
176. Smith, P., Lee, M.: Cross-discourse development of supervised sentiment analysis in the clinical domain. In: Proceedings of the 3rd Workshop in Computational Approaches to Subjectivity and Sentiment Analysis, pp. 79–83 (2012)
177. Smuha, N.A.: The EU approach to ethics guidelines for trustworthy artificial intelligence. Comput. Law Rev. Int. **20**(4), 97–106 (2019)
178. Socher, R., Perelygin, A., Wu, J., Chuang, J., Manning, C.D., Ng, A.Y., Potts, C.: Recursive deep models for semantic compositionality over a sentiment treebank. In: Proceedings of the 2013 Conference on Empirical Methods in Natural Language Processing, pp. 1631–1642 (2013)
179. Sohn, S., Torii, M., Li, D., Wagholikar, K.B., Wu, S.T.I., Liu, H.: A hybrid approach to sentiment sentence classification in suicide notes. Biomed. Inf. Insights **5**, 43–50 (2012)
180. Spasić, I., Burnap, P., Greenwood, M., Arribas-Ayllon, M.: A naïve Bayes approach to classifying topics in suicide notes. Biomed. Inf. Insights **5**, BII–S8945 (2012)
181. Spasić, I., Owen, D., Smith, A., Button, K.: Klosure: closing in on open–ended patient questionnaires with text mining. J. Biomed. Semantics **10**(1), 1–11 (2019)
182. Strapparava, C., Valitutti, A., et al.: Wordnet affect: an affective extension of wordnet. In: Lrec, vol. 4, p. 40. Lisbon (2004)
183. Straw, I.: Ethical implications of emotion mining in medicine. Health Pol. Technol. **10**(1), 191–195 (2021)
184. Stubbs, A., Kotfila, C., Xu, H., Uzuner, Ö: Identifying risk factors for heart disease over time: overview of 2014 i2b2/uthealth shared task track 2. J. Biomed. Inf. **58**, S67–S77 (2015). https://doi.org/10.1016/j.jbi.2015.07.001. http://www.sciencedirect.com/science/article/pii/S1532046415001409. Proceedings of the 2014 i2b2/UTHealth Shared-Tasks and Workshop on Challenges in Natural Language Processing for Clinical Data
185. Subirats, L., Conesa, J., Armayones, M.: Biomedical holistic ontology for people with rare diseases. Int. J. Environ. Res. Public Health **17**(17), 6038 (2020)
186. Sun, Q., Tang, T.Y.: On the computational study of Chinese Alzheimer's disease online communities: a sentiment and contextual analysis approach. In: Proceedings of the International Conference on Pattern Recognition and Artificial Intelligence, pp. 104–108 (2018). https://doi.org/10.1145/3243250.3243259
187. Takats, C., Kwan, A., Wormer, R., Goldman, D., Jones, H.E., Romero, D., et al.: Ethical and methodological considerations of twitter data for public health research: systematic review. J. Med. Internet Res. **24**(11), e40380 (2022)

188. Tanushi, H., Dalianis, H., Duneld, M., Kvist, M., Skeppstedt, M., Velupillai, S.: Negation scope delimitation in clinical text using three approaches: Negex, pycontextnlp and synneg. In: 19th Nordic Conference of Computational Linguistics (NODALIDA 2013), May 22-24, 2013, Oslo, pp. 387–474. Linköping University Electronic Press (2013)
189. Tausczik, Y.R., Pennebaker, J.W.: The psychological meaning of words: Liwc and computerized text analysis methods. J. Lang. Soc. Psychol. **29**(1), 24–54 (2010)
190. Tsao, S.F., MacLean, A., Chen, H., Li, L., Yang, Y., Butt, Z.A.: Public attitudes during the second lockdown: sentiment and topic analyses using tweets from Ontario, Canada. Int. J. Public Health **67**, 1604658 (2022)
191. Turcan, E., Muresan, S., McKeown, K.: Emotion-infused models for explainable psychological stress detection. In: Proceedings of the 2021 Conference of the North American Chapter of the Association for Computational Linguistics: Human Language Technologies, pp. 2895–2909. Association for Computational Linguistics, Online (2021). https://doi.org/10.18653/v1/2021.naacl-main.230. https://aclanthology.org/2021.naacl-main.230
192. Uban, A.S., Chulvi, B., Rosso, P.: An emotion and cognitive based analysis of mental health disorders from social media data. Future Gener. Comput. Syst. **124**, 480–494 (2021)
193. Uzuner, Ö.: Recognizing obesity and comorbidities in sparse data. J. Am. Med. Inf. Assoc. **16**(4), 561–570 (2009). https://doi.org/10.1197/jamia.M3115
194. Walonoski, J., Kramer, M., Nichols, J., Quina, A., Moesel, C., Hall, D., Duffett, C., Dube, K., Gallagher, T., McLachlan, S.: Synthea: an approach, method, and software mechanism for generating synthetic patients and the synthetic electronic health care record. J. Am. Med. Inf. Assoc. **25**(3), 230–238 (2018)
195. Wang, Y., McKee, M., Torbica, A., Stuckler, D.: Systematic literature review on the spread of health-related misinformation on social media. Soc. Sci. Med. **240**, 112552 (2019)
196. Wang, Y., Zhao, Y., Zhang, J., Bian, J., Zhang, R.: Detecting associations between dietary supplement intake and sentiments within mental disorder tweets. Health Inf. J. **26**(2), 803–815 (2020)
197. Warren, J., Tempero, E., Warren, I., Sathianathan, A., Hopkins, S., Shepherd, M., Merry, S.: Experience building it infrastructure for research with online youth mental health tools. In: 2018 25th Australasian Software Engineering Conference (ASWEC), pp. 161–165. IEEE (2018)
198. Waudby-Smith, I.E., Tran, N., Dubin, J.A., Lee, J.: Sentiment in nursing notes as an indicator of out-of-hospital mortality in intensive care patients. PloS One **13**(6), e0198687 (2018)
199. Weissman, G.E., Ungar, L.H., Harhay, M.O., Courtright, K.R., Halpern, S.D.: Construct validity of six sentiment analysis methods in the text of encounter notes of patients with critical illness. J. Biomed. Inf. **89**, 114–121 (2019)
200. Wild, C.P.: Complementing the genome with an "exposome": the outstanding challenge of environmental exposure measurement in molecular epidemiology. Cancer Epidemiol. Biomark. Prevention **14**(8), 1847–1850 (2005)
201. Wilkins, C.H.: Effective engagement requires trust and being trustworthy. Med. Care **56**, S6–S8 (2018)
202. Wu, H., Lu, N.: Service provision, pricing, and patient satisfaction in online health communities. Int. J. Med. Inf. **110**, 77–89 (2018)
203. Xue, W., Li, T.: Aspect based sentiment analysis with gated convolutional networks. In: Proceedings of the 56th Annual Meeting of the Association for Computational Linguistics (Volume 1: Long Papers), pp. 2514–2523. Association for Computational Linguistics, Melbourne (2018). https://doi.org/10.18653/v1/P18-1234. https://www.aclweb.org/anthology/P18-1234
204. Yadav, S., Ekbal, A., Saha, S., Bhattacharyya, P.: Medical sentiment analysis using social media: towards building a patient assisted system. In: Proceedings of the Eleventh International Conference on Language Resources and Evaluation (LREC 2018) (2018)
205. Yoo, M., Jang, C.W.: Physical rehabilitation on social media during covid-19: topics and sentiments analysis of tweets. Ann. Phys. Rehab. Med. **65**, 101589–101589 (2021)

206. Yu, K.H., Kohane, I.S.: Framing the challenges of artificial intelligence in medicine. BMJ Qual. Saf. **28**(3), 238–241 (2019)
207. Zhang, Y., Zhao, Z., Wang, P., Li, X., Rong, L., Song, D.: InteractiveSentimentDataset. IEEE Dataport (2020). https://doi.org/10.21227/d3rf-sd41
208. Zhang, Y., Zhao, Z., Wang, P., Li, X., Rong, L., Song, D.: Scenariosa: a dyadic conversational database for interactive sentiment analysis. IEEE Access **8**, 90652–90664 (2020). https://doi.org/10.1109/ACCESS.2020.2994147
209. Zhang, Z., Hamadi, H.A., Damiani, E., Yeun, C.Y., Taher, F.: Explainable artificial intelligence applications in cyber security: state-of-the-art in research. Preprint. arXiv:2208.14937 (2022)
210. Zou Y., Wang J., Lei Z., Zhang Y., Wang W.: Sentiment analysis for necessary preview of 30-day mortality in sepsis patients and the control strategies. J. Healthc. Eng. **2021**, Article 1713363 (2021). https://doi.org/10.1155/2021/1713363
211. Zucco, C., Liang, H., Fatta, G.D., Cannataro, M.: Explainable sentiment analysis with applications in medicine. In: 2018 IEEE International Conference on Bioinformatics and Biomedicine (BIBM), pp. 1740–1747 (2018). https://doi.org/10.1109/BIBM.2018.8621359
212. Zunic, A., Corcoran, P., Spasic, I., et al.: Sentiment analysis in health and well-being: systematic review. JMIR Med. Inf. **8**(1), e16023 (2020)

Index

K. Denecke, *Sentiment Analysis in the Medical Domain*,
https://doi.org/10.1007/978-3-031-30187-2

V